MOVE WITH BALANCE®

MOVE WITH BALANCE®

HEALTHY AGING ACTIVITIES
FOR BRAIN AND BODY

KAREN PETERSON, M.A.

FOREWORD BY EDVIN MANNIKO, O.D.

Giving Back® Books

Pa'ia, Hawai'i

Published by
Giving Back®
Pa'ia, Hawai'i

ISBN-10 0985993804
ISBN-13 978-0-9859938-0-1

Library of Congress Control Number: 2012951095

Editor: Paul Wood
Cover and Book Design: Karen Bacon
Photography: David Watersun (the movements)
            Karen Peterson, Peggy Sanches, James Mylenek (candid shots)

Giving Back® and Move With Balance® are trademarked by Karen Peterson, executive director of
Giving Back®, a Hawai'i nonprofit corporation.
www.GivingBackMentoring.org
www.MoveWithBalance.org

To Gammy

ELDER CREED

"An elder is a person who is still growing, still a learner, still with potential and whose life continues to have within it promise for, and connection to, the future. An elder is still in pursuit of happiness, joy, and pleasure, and her or his birthright to these remains intact. Moreover, an elder is a person who deserves respect and honor and whose work it is to synthesize wisdom from long life experience and formulate this into a legacy for future generations."

~Zalman Shalomi-Schacter

Contents

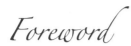

Foreword

Visual skills are developed from birth and learned as the individual grows. They can also be taught, enhanced, and improved at any age. The visual system is a complex process that involves the mind, muscles, eyes, and subtle, complicated mechanisms that tie everything together—it's much more than just acuity (i.e., 20/20 vision).

Visual therapy involves this entire visual system—representing a form of neurological training or rehabilitation. It can be compared to some forms of occupational therapy or physical therapy. The overriding goal of the therapy is to train the patient's brain to use the eyes to receive information effectively, comprehend it quickly, and react appropriately.

More than eighty percent of all sensory information is derived from the visual system. Improving the visual system can significantly boost performance by improving response time, vision-body coordination, and confidence.

Vision is an active and dynamic process. What we see is influenced by more than just the light-signals sent to our eyes from the world around us. Vision also consists of visual and motor signals, our ability to move our eyes, and the attention we bring to bear on an object. Research has shown that we actually do not see many things in our environment simply because we are not paying attention to them.

Seniors who fall are often seriously hurt, and that damage leads to undesirable consequences. But the human balance system is trainable for children, athletes, and seniors. Twenty percent of the information going to the eyes ends up in the balance system. (To prove this try to balance with your eyes closed.)

I met Karen Peterson twenty-five years ago when she introduced me to her expertise in movement and perception. We worked together to help alleviate vision and balance issues. Her present concern is enhancing balance and thereby preventing falls. This program is based on cutting-edge science. She uses modified techniques that Olympic athletes employ with good success.

I wholeheartedly endorse her work to make seniors safer and to help them lead more active and productive lives.

Sincerely,
Edvin Manniko, O.D.

Our Story

Karen Peterson founded and directs Giving Back, a nonprofit organization dedicated to improving the lives of elders through intergenerational mentoring. She is a licensed Brain Gym® instructor, a certified educational kinesiologist, a certified natural vision improvement instructor, a certified Touch for Health instructor, and a certified massage therapist. Since 1987 she has been teaching these modalities to children, businesspeople, athletes, classroom teachers, and adults of all ages and occupations.

In 1994 she began teaching movement exercises to senior citizens in her home community of Maui, Hawai'i. She believes that elders are a vitally important resource and need to be integrated into the fabric of our society. One of her early innovations was to launch a program that brought elders and children together at a local elementary school for "intergenerational mentoring." Inspired by the program's success, in 2000 she created Giving Back, a nonprofit agency whose intergenerational programs provide a structured way for senior citizens to "give back" to their communities.

In 2005 she expanded the program such that active elders began mentoring frail elders. In every case this mentoring involved using healthy, centering activities that she derived from her diverse professional training. Those activities, tested and clarified through innumerable sessions by hundreds of volunteers, are presented here in this manual.

Karen's elder-to-elder approach evolved into Move With Balance®, a healthy-aging program that helps prevent falls, enhances cognitive skills, and improves the quality of life for all participants. In March 2012 she was flown to Washington D.C. to attend the National Forum on Brain Health at the American Society on Aging Conference, where she was honored with the 2012 Metlife MindAlert Award in the Mental Fitness General category. In March 2010 Mutual of America Foundation presented Move With Balance® an award of $15,000 for the purpose of replicating its practices through print and digital publication. What began as one determined woman working in a small island community has grown into a nationally recognized program focused on enhanced quality of life for senior citizens everywhere.

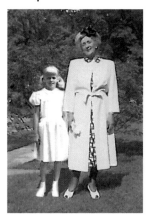

She says, "When I turned fifty, I started to feel younger. I wanted to 'give back,' to be of service. At the time I was teaching senior citizens, and I saw how vibrant and full of wisdom most of them were. I was sure that others of my generation would want to share their gifts, enthusiasm, and vitality with their communities, especially with those older and less vigorous than they. My inspiration for all this work has been the memory of my own grandmother, Gammy. We bonded closely, and she became an important mentor for me."

Our Unique Solution

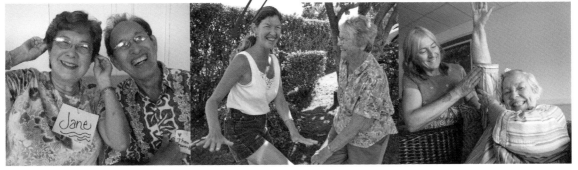

Welcome!

Welcome to Move With Balance®, a program that will improve your well-being and the well-being of the elders you serve. This book and the videos demonstrate movements that enhance any person's sense of balance and improve cognitive functions but they are especially geared to elders. Their effect is proven to be rejuvenating, even life-saving, for people in their late-life years.

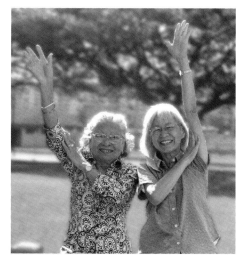

This program is designed to enhance whole-brain integration and to develop a strong connection between the body and the brain. Its goal is to change the elder's physiology and nervous system on a very deep level.

And to have fun doing so.

We focus on vision training and sensory motor integration. Our methods include strengthening exercises for the lower body, regular balance exercises, and other integrative, fun activities and games that progressively challenge the elder's balance and brain in a safe environment.

People take the sense of balance for granted—until the day comes when they slip, lose control, and fall. But each of us can prevent such an event by realizing that balance is a skill. With practice this skill can be developed and maintained.

The Move With Balance® activities facilitate eye-brain-body connections through specific movement experiences. They promote efficient communication among the many nerve cells and functional centers in sensory motor system. They free our innate ability to learn and function at top efficiency.

Proven Benefits

One independent evaluation of Move With Balance® shows improvement in lower and upper body strength, aerobic endurance, lower and upper body flexibility, agility, and dynamic balance in older adults. Another independent evaluation shows improvement in balance during sitting, standing, and walking activities of older adults, not to mention overall improved mental, physical, and emotional well-being.

In our most recent independent evaluation (June 2012) our objective was to compare the number of falls in the exercising group to the number of falls in those serving as controls (no exercise). Although the study is in the process of being published for peer review, we can say that there was a statistically significant reduction in falls in our target group—38 percent fewer!

See Appendix D for summaries of these evaluations. Full evaluations are available on www.MoveWithBalance.org.

Vision: Much More Than Seeing

Vision gives the nervous system updated information about the position of body parts in relation to each other and the environment. With that information we judge distances, avoid obstacles, and control our balance. Good depth perception enables us to judge terrain and distances. Without good depth perception we experience eyestrain, fatigue, headaches, balance and posture problems, and memory loss. Move With Balance® is all about improving visual/motor performance by training both eyes and the brain to coordinate. We call that smooth-running state "fusion."

We see in two ways. The most familiar way of seeing is right through the macula of the eye's retina—20/20 vision. But we also get lots of important information through our peripheral vision. For example, even when we spot a hundred-dollar-bill in the gutter, we remain aware of the traffic around us. Peripheral vision is primarily a spatial orientation system.

Nerve fibers from the peripheral retina go directly to the midbrain, where they become part of the sensory motor pathway. These images inform our kinesthetic, proprioceptive, vestibular, and tactile systems, which are crucial for orientation and movement. In other words, they help us know and control where we are in space. When people get old, they tend to lose their control of this seeing-based system that provides spatial orientation.

Movement is the Answer

Paul Dennison of Brain Gym International® and the Educational Kinesiology Foundation says, "Movement is the door to learning." When we move in new and different ways, the brain changes. It naturally develops new skills.

Move With Balance® brings integrated new ways of moving to the elders. At first, the movements may be slow and difficult for them. Their nervous systems feel a sense of chaos while they are learning. But after they have practiced and repeated the movements, new neural pathways are laid down. The now-improved brain puts those movements on automatic pilot. Change has taken place.

At any age we can still learn balance, how to be grounded, how to know where we are in space, how to stay centered and aware, how to feel the brain/body connection.

OUR WONDERFUL BRAINS

The term "brain plasticity" refers to the brain's ability to change and grow. Michael Merzenich M.D. and Ph.D. (University of California at San Francisco), one of the leading researchers in this field, says that the brain is not static. As long as it is alive, it responds to new learning and new circumstances. Brain plasticity is a physical process that manifests as changes in our abilities. As new neural pathways grow, the brain is rewired and we move in new ways with new abilities.

THE GOAL

Our movements, performed in the manner described, will strengthen the integration of the sensory-motor and the vestibular systems of all who perform them, no matter what

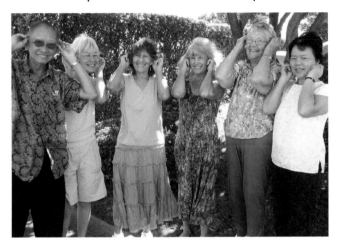

the age. Elders become more present in their bodies. They know where they are in space. They are balanced from the inside out—from their nervous systems to their physical surroundings. Their whole brains are activated. They become more confident in their movements, moving with ease and comfort.

Then they become willing to exercise beyond the program.

ALL TOGETHER NOW

Our culture expects older people to decline, not move—to be "set in their ways" and not try new things. But research has shown that the brain learns and changes throughout our lives. We have to exercise our brains to keep them growing.

This is best done by coordinated movement—activities that combine movement with cognitive skills. For example, in Move With Balance® we move, but while we move we read, or recognize shapes, or recite a poem. Ideally, in a single activity we stimulate many senses—for example, visual, auditory, and kinesthetic at the same time. The underlying principle: challenge the brain and body simultaneously with some sensory-motor activity, repeat until the challenge becomes easier or even automatic, then up the stakes by repeating the activity at a higher level.

Our Aging Population: Some Alarming Statistics

Falls

The National Council on Aging reports that every year one in three US citizens aged 65 and older takes a spill. Every eighteen seconds an old person comes to some hospital emergency room needing treatment for having lost balance and hit the ground. Every 35 minutes some elder dies from the complications following such a tumble. In fact, falling is the leading cause of injury-related death among people age 65 and older. In 2005 falls accounted for almost 16,000 fatalities.

We spend more than $19 billion each year to treat injuries from falls. The average hospitalization for such injuries costs $17,500. By 2020, the annual costs for fall-related injuries are expected to reach $54.9 billion (in 2007 dollars).

And yet research shows us that most falls are preventable.

Mild Cognitive Impairment

Age-related cognitive decline is a huge problem. The disorder known as Mild Cognitive Impairment (MCI) afflicts ten to twenty percent of older adults in the US and in four Western European countries.

Ronald Peterson, neurologist and director of the Mayo Clinic Alzheimer's Disease Research Center, reports that "If we consider the sixteen percent prevalence of mild cognitive impairment in individuals without dementia, then add the ten to eleven percent of individuals who already have dementia or Alzheimer's disease, we're looking at 25 percent or more of the population aged seventy or older who have dementia or are at risk of developing dementia in the near future. With the aging of America, these numbers are staggering. The impact on the health-care economy, as well as on individuals and their families, is quite impressive. The need for early diagnosis and therapeutic intervention is increasingly important."

Enhancing Balance

The following passage comes from the book *Physical Activities for Improving Children's Behavior* written by Billye Ann Cheatum, a Ph.D. in physical and special education, and Alison A. Hammond, a sensory motor development specialist:

"Vestibular input is necessary for static and dynamic balance development, eye-tracking ability, and motor planning. Children who are slow to develop vestibular functioning are delayed in all gross motor patterns, which require coordination of both sides of the body. They may have difficulty in maintaining posture with eye-hand coordination, and with fine motor control."

In Move With Balance® we work directly with the vestibular system, stimulating and integrating it with the visual, auditory, and kinesthetic systems in order to give balance and focus to elders. You should know, though, that many of the movements described in this manual were developed for use with children. For years, we used most of these same exercises in an intergenerational mentoring program in which active seniors mentored children, helping them with their concentration and coordination. Our experience shows us that these movements benefit anyone who practices them, no matter what age.

Improving Cognitive Skills: Growing the Brain

In the preface to her second edition of *Smart Moves: Why Learning Is Not All In Your Head* (Great River Books) Dr. Carla Hannaford writes, "Today, it seems, we are finally coming

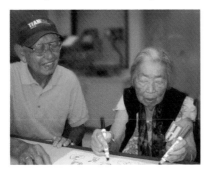

to grasp that movement and sensory experiences are the fertile soil for continued brain development and growth for a lifetime—and that those experiences actually cause the brain to constantly transform itself in unimaginably plastic ways."

In other words, our brains can continue to grow and learn. It is not inevitable that they shrink and falter. How exciting it is to hear a scientist confirm what Move With Balance® has been demonstrating all along—that by practicing simple activities, many of them the sort of games we played as children, we can increase the brain's agility and keep on going. By growing.

You can find an in-depth essay on this topic by Dr. Hannaford in Appendix E.

Getting Started

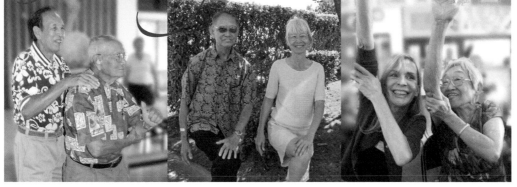

MEMBERSHIP

In addition to this book, we have many videos on the website. Once you buy the book, you have access to the videos. The book explains the movements in depth, the why and the how. The videos give you a quick visual, and in combination with the book they make it easy for you to learn the movements. Our website (MoveWithBalance.org) offers further resources. These include all the Activity Cards from Appendix B, new activities, helpful supplies, and news from the world of elder care. As you get more involved with the program, you'll want to consider an online membership. Our intention is to create an online community of members who share and interact. This will organically develop. Once the web community grows, we will give you access to a widespread and growing community through webinars, access to experts in the field, interactive blogs, and other forms of networking. As a member, you will also find how-to coaching for extending this work along one of three application models.

APPLICATION MODELS

GROUP LEADER MODEL

Our entire program evolved through the application of this kind of service. For someone with the enthusiasm and passion to help elders, the decision to lead groups has proven to be deeply satisfying. Opportunities for such positive applications are everywhere. They include senior centers and housing complexes, lunch sites, exercise rooms, assisted living facilities, outpatient rehabilitation facilities, hospitals, nursing homes, and adult daycare centers. We can show you how to design a group program by recruiting and training active seniors, who in turn volunteer as one-to-one mentors of frail elders. The group leader becomes the facilitator, leading the activities while the mentors individualize the activities for the frail elders in a safe, loving environment. All participants experience enhanced balance, vision, coordination, and cognitive function.

Our website provides aspiring group leaders with plenty of help and encouragement—a Group Leader Manual, news and webinars, answers to specific questions, but most of all the connection to a community of like-minded people who feel the value of this work.

PROFESSIONAL CAREGIVER MODEL

Move With Balance® speaks to any organization or individual who works one-on-one with elders—caregiver agencies, individual professionals, and physical therapists, for example. Skilled professionals can adapt the Move With Balance® program to the needs and constraints of any single therapeutic session. Our interactive website gives access to the professional community through blogs and webinars, guest speakers, articles and updates. Let us help you add a new dimension to your one-on-one sessions, progressive and simple activities that are proven by scientific research to improve the health of your client.

PERSONAL MODEL

The Move With Balance® activities are perfectly designed for solo use at any age, particularly all mobile, independent seniors who want to improve their balance, vision, coordination, and cognitive functions. Experience has taught us, however, that working with a partner or a group of friends will add zest and consistency to the discipline of regular practice. Friendly, caring interaction is itself a form of therapy.

Either way, our website provides members with a network intended to support the involvement of individuals. Through our online assistance you can get hold of the simple equipment useful for certain activities. You can attend webinars, hear guest speakers, read blogs and newsletters, learn new exercises, and experience being part of a community that is dedicated to staying in balance for life.

DESIGNING A SESSION

AN ART, NOT A FORMULA

Each activity in this manual includes an approximate implementation time. But we would be wrong to prescribe a set format or timetable for session designs. Elders are remarkably diverse in their mental and physical skills. The planning and leading of sessions is a kind of art form that draws on the powers of observation, compassion, and intuition.

At first you will need to go slowly. You and your partner, group, or client are learning. The time you spend on any one activity might exceed the time stated in the description. That is perfectly fine. Once the exercises become more familiar and the participants learn their own skill levels, you will naturally pick up the pace. Strive for balance between the time available and the skills of all involved.

Your primary job is to keep challenging the elders (and yourself) in ways that are always fun. The brain loves what is novel and difficult. That's when we grow new brain cells, regain our balance, and more. So start with sitting, then move to standing, and then walking. When participants master an activity, progress. Make the activity more challenging.

This program is extraordinarily adaptable. You get a wide range of activities to choose from, so you'll want to change, mix it up, and experiment. Each activity includes simple ways to keep boosting the challenge. As soon as any one activity gets easy or routine, change. Challenge means growth, and that's what we want—growth of the brain and the integrated neural systems that keep us on our toes.

Some participants get frustrated with this experience of ever-increasing challenge. They want to "get there" and "win the game." That's why it is so important to keep the spirit of play in everything. Think of kids during school recess. Whatever they're doing with such admirable enthusiasm—jumping rope, playing rhythmic hand games, or dodging a ball—they do it to the edge of their abilities, then fail, then start again. Their unstated question is "How well can I do this tricky thing today, and how much better will I get at it tomorrow?" On the psychological level, Move With Balance® is a lot about reminding old people to act like kids. To play.

If you take a leadership role in this work, your goal will be to inspire maximum performance improvement for each elder in each session. Talking, listening, paying attention, experimenting, and laughing—these are all part of the process. By the way, this kind of leadership is good for the leader, too.

A Typical One-Hour Session

Warm Up—approximately 15 minutes
Lengthening muscles, getting present, brain/body integration, waking up the senses. Now you're ready to go.

More-Active Exercises—approximately 15-20 minutes
Cross-Crawl, You the Dancer, Balls, Beanbags, Childhood Games, Strengthen Your Legs, Vision and Balance

Integration Time—approximately 5 minutes
Pause and bring the senses into harmony.

Less Active Exercises—approximately 15-20 minutes
Confidence Walk, Focus on Your Feet, Sensory Integration, Sharpen Your Vision with Fusion.

Integration Time—approximately 5 minutes
Rest and relax.

Traditionally we end each session with the Gandhi Farewell (page 68). After that you might want to use the self-reporting inventories that you'll find in Appendix C (or on our website). These forms and questionnaires are useful if you wish to show evidence of improvement, for example to a donor or senior-living facility. They are not necessary for the activities to be effective.

This describes a typical one-hour session. But you can do a fifteen-minute session, too. Again, you should experiment and find your way of applying the activities to your unique situation.

MORE COACHING

POSTURE

Improving your posture improves your health, your breathing, and your balance. Be conscious of your posture when doing all the Move With Balance® activities. Stand tall, shoulders back. Keep your head up and your eyes forward. Have confidence.

WATER

Your body is sixty to seventy percent water. Blood is mostly water, and your muscles, lungs, and brain all contain a lot of water. Your body needs water to regulate body temperature and to provide the means for nutrients to travel to all your organs. Water also transports oxygen to your cells, removes waste, and protects your joints and organs

Drink plenty of water during the activities. Drinking water helps keep the brain sufficiently hydrated. Since the brain is also a vast series of electrical impulses—and water helps to conduct electricity—it is obvious that drinking water will assist the brain in thinking clearly. Water provides energy for the electrical activities in the brain.

BREATHING

Breathe continuously through each activity. Notice and check yourself often to see if you are breathing. When under stress, we tend to hold our breath. When breathing is shallow, the lower section of the lungs does not fill with oxygen, and this holding-back limits the oxygen supply. When breathing is full, there is an abundant supply of oxygen to nourish the brain.

We can use breathing consciously to influence the involuntary (sympathetic) nervous system that regulates blood pressure, heart rate, circulation, digestion, and many other bodily functions.

Try this: while you do the movements, imagine that you have a cord coming out of you that you plug into a socket. Then you become a breathing machine.

SAFETY

Make sure you carefully watch, protect, and keep the frail elders safe. Hang onto the back of a chair or be near a wall when doing the movements. Adapt the movements to the abilities of the senior.

THE PROGRESSIVE CHALLENGE

The brain loves to learn, enjoying what is new and fresh. As soon as you can do the activity, go to the next level. Mix things up. Keep progressing and challenging.

COGNITIVE TASKS

The movement descriptions indicate where it might be beneficial to add a cognitive task, such as doing simple math problems, counting backwards, saying the alphabet backwards, spelling your name backwards, reading an eye chart, or having a conversation.

DROPPING IN

This is the ultimate goal. Some call this "rooting" or "noticing." When we say "dropping in," we mean the experience of getting completely secure within your body. There's no disconnect or blurry lack of physical presence. You feel yourself inside your body. You are present with all the movements. You notice what you are doing. You are aware.

Dropping in will strengthen the brain-body connection.

STRESS

Watch for signs of stress, such as shortness of breath, other changes in breathing, sweating, dizziness, loss of focus, disorientation, nausea, change in face color, pain, or sudden fatigue. If you notice such responses, stop the movement and take a break. Go to the Integration Time: Rest and Relax section. Do the Emotional Stress Release activity (see page 66).

The Movements

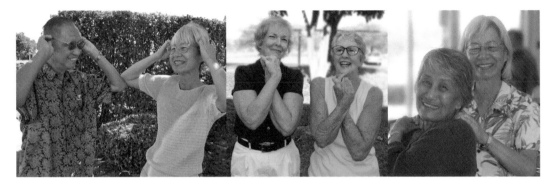

WARM-UPS

Always warm up for five to ten minutes before an extended activity session. Pick from any of the warm-ups described below. It's not necessary to do them all every time. But we suggest that you mix them up with the intent of sampling them all over a period of time.

The first six warm-ups are adapted from the Brain Gym® repertoire. The next three were inspired by Touch For Health.

ARM ACTIVATION (4 MIN)

Why:

Arm Activation lengthens the muscles of the upper chest and shoulders, the origin of muscular control for fine and gross motor activities. When gross-motor tension is released, fine motor skills are enhanced. Arm Activation helps release the feeling of "carrying the world on our shoulders." With fewer burdens, you can be more present to enjoy life. Use this activity to improve posture, hand-eye coordination, writing, and penmanship.

How:

- ◆ Hold one arm straight up next to the ear.
- ◆ Place opposite hand on the upper arm.
- ◆ Remember to keep breathing in a relaxed, easy way.
- ◆ Push the arm against the hand and the hand against the arm.
- ◆ Use some strength. Use your muscles. Imagine that your arm is a wall and you are pushing your hand against it.
- ◆ Repeat by pushing, one by one, in all four directions: forward, backward, then towards and away from the ear.
- ◆ Notice the difference of feeling between muscle activation and muscle relaxation.
- ◆ After completing one side, notice how relaxed the activated shoulder feels compared to the opposite shoulder. Put both arms straight out in front of you. Notice that the arm you activated is longer!
- ◆ Switch arms and repeat the entire sequence on the other side. Check that arms are both the same length.

LAZY 8S (5 MIN)

Why:

Have you ever read a page from a book and had no idea what it said? The left hemisphere of the brain controls vision for the right eye, and the right hemisphere controls vision for the left eye. When the two hemispheres work together as a team, visual perception is clear and integrated. Then, reading is easy. So is balance. Depth perception improves balance.

How:

The "8" is called "lazy" because the shape you draw is flopped horizontal rather than vertical—"∞ ." It's the infinity symbol, a circular crossing and recrossing of the mid-line of your body.

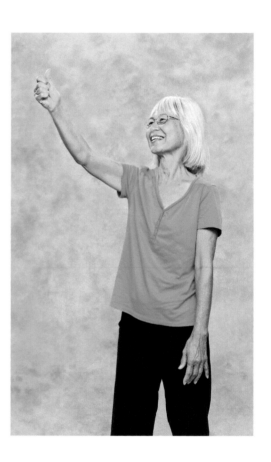

Left arm:

◆ Extend the arm directly forward with the thumb pointing up.

◆ Focus the eyes softly on the thumbnail.

◆ Lazily move the thumb to trace the ∞ (infinity) shape in the air. Start at the midpoint of the ∞, moving up to the left or to the right, then around, then moving up through the midpoint again and around.

◆ Always up through the midpoint.

◆ Keep your head stationary, and let both your eyes easily follow the thumbnail.

◆ Stay relaxed. Repeat several times.

Right arm:

◆ Repeat the sequence as with left arm.

Both arms:

◆ Repeat with both arms extended, hands together thumbs up.

◆ Same pattern. Upward motion at the midpoint, either way.

◆ Notice if the eyes can easily see all the parts of movement. If any area is out of focus or unseen, slow down until the brain learns to see it.

THE ELEPHANT (5 MIN)

Why:

The Elephant integrates listening for both ears as it releases tight neck muscles. It enhances eye-teaming ability. You are crossing the auditory mid-line and thus refreshing the skills of attention, recognition, perception, discrimination, and memory. This activity enhances short- and long-term memory as well as silent speech and thinking ability. Use it to integrate vision, listening, and whole-body movement. It activates the inner ear to sharpen your sense of balance.

How:

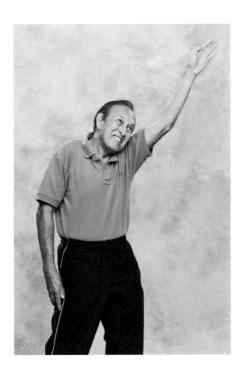

Left arm:

- ◆ Stand with knees comfortably bent.
- ◆ Stretch out your left arm, fingers extended.
- ◆ Lay your head on your left shoulder. Think of the arm as your elephant trunk. It's as if the head is glued to the shoulder. Keep both eyes open and looking easily at your fingertips.
- ◆ Now trace the Lazy 8 (the previous activity), this time by moving from your waist. Sway as though are an elephant, relaxed and content.
- ◆ Always up through the midpoint.
- ◆ Torso, head, and arm function as one unit. No body-twist is involved.
- ◆ Do this several times.

Right arm:

- ◆ Stretch out your right arm, fingers extended.
- ◆ Head on right shoulder.
- ◆ Repeat the Lazy 8 as with left arm.
- ◆ Do this several times.

Easier Variations:

- ◆ Instead of Lazy 8, trace a rainbow, an arc back and forth.
- ◆ Do The Elephant while sitting.

THE OWL (4 MIN)

Why:

This neck-and-shoulder activity releases tension in the upper trapezius muscles. It enhances auditory skills and improves focus and attention. Blinking relaxes visual skills. The "whoooo" sound relaxes auditory/listening skills.

The Owl promotes focus and concentration. Use it when you find your focus distracted by endless thoughts or auditory sounds. It improves communication and helps you listen more effectively. It helps with spelling and the ability to access visual memory and auditory constructs. It improves posture.

How:

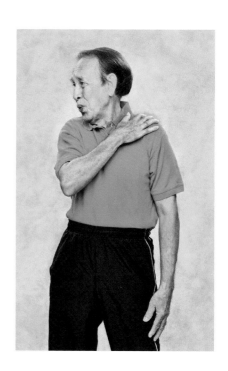

- ◆ With the right hand, grasp the left shoulder muscle near the neck.
- ◆ Turn your head to look at your right hand holding your left shoulder.
- ◆ Inhale and squeeze the muscle firmly.
- ◆ Now exhale as you rotate your head to the right side to look back over the right shoulder. Continue to inhale and exhale during the rotation.
- ◆ Make an owl-like "whooooo" sound as you exhale. Blink.
- ◆ Do this several times.
- ◆ Then drop your chin to your chest while relaxing your shoulder muscle.
- ◆ Repeat, using the left hand on the right shoulder.

THE FOOT FLEX (4 MIN)

Why:

The calf muscle is one of the first parts of the body to respond to danger. Its posture of withdrawal, called the tendon guard reflex, is a common physiological reaction to stress and overload. Tension in the calf can translate into tension in the lower back and then in the neck. Holding the calf muscle in the lengthened position while moving the foot back and forth teaches the brain to release that tension. By relaxing this muscle, you gain better posture and a centered, relaxed view on the world.

Use The Foot Flex to ease tension in communicating with others. It helps you express yourself clearly, both orally and in writing. It helps you align your body for good posture and better balance.

How:

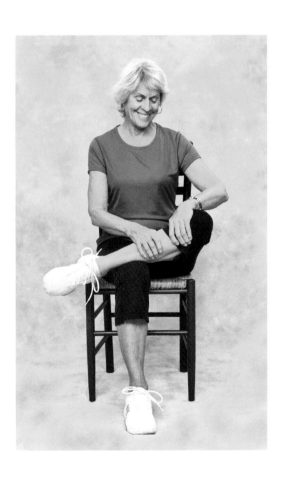

- While sitting, cross one leg over the other, placing the ankle on the opposite the knee.

- Place your thumbs in the meaty part of the calf muscle and feel for sore spots.

- Also check the ankle and beneath the knee.

- While holding the sore spots, alternate pointing and flexing the foot.

- Use the ankle to make circles with the foot, clockwise and counterclockwise, while holding sore points with your thumbs.

- Repeat with the other leg.

- After, notice the lengthening of the calf muscle.

- Notice the increased range of the point and flex.

- Stand and notice that your knees are relaxed and not locked.

- You can do The Foot Flex lying down. Many have said this activity helps to eliminate leg cramps at night.

THE GRAVITY GLIDER (5-8 MIN)

Why:

When you reach forward from the ribcage, the legs and back muscles lengthen and relax. Tension in the hips and pelvis gets released. This frees you to sit and stand in more comfortable postures. This activity improves reading comprehension and abstract thinking. It gives a sense of grounding and centering, balance and coordination. It enhances confidence and stability along with self-expression.

How:

- ◆ Sit comfortably, crossing one ankle over the other.
- ◆ Bend forward, reaching towards your feet.
- ◆ Let gravity draw your hands down to the right side of your feet.
- ◆ Hang like a rag doll.
- ◆ Inhale and exhale, feeling your spine rise and fall as you reach down.
- ◆ Slowly come up with your back rounded, bringing your head up last.
- ◆ Breathe. Notice your straight spine.
- ◆ Bend forward as before, but this time reach toward the left side of your feet.
- ◆ Hang like a rag doll, then as before slowly come up.
- ◆ Bend forward as before, but this time reach down to the center of your crossed ankles.
- ◆ Hang like a rag doll, then as before slowly come up.
- ◆ Cross your feet the other way and repeat the activity, right, left, and center.
- ◆ Always come up slowly with rounded back, head last.
- ◆ Always breathe deeply and move slowly.
- ◆ With your ankles crossed, experiment with having your feet flat on the floor and then having only the heels on the floor.

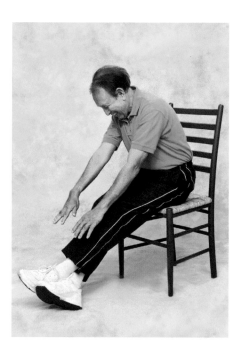

Shorter Variation:

- ◆ Cross ankles and reach down the center only. Come up.
- ◆ Cross ankles the other way and reach down the center. Come up.

WAKE UP (3 MIN)

Why:

The kinesthetic stimulation takes place just above where the two carotid arteries branch as they leave the heart, carrying freshly oxygenated blood to the brain. The hand on the navel brings attention to the gravitational center of the body, where the core muscles contribute to balance. This activity stimulates neuro-lymphatic reflex points and acts like a light switch, allowing increased energy throughout the body. Do this when you want to wake up, be alert, and focus clearly. This activity helps with whole-body coordination.

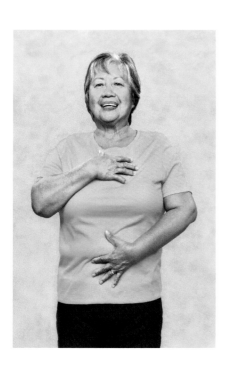

How:

♦ Using both hands, massage and stimulate the points between your first and second ribs, directly under the collar bone, to the right and left of your sternum.

♦ Massage deeply for twenty to thirty seconds until any tenderness is released.

♦ Then place one hand over the navel while the other hand holds the points you just stimulated.

♦ Switch hands.

Variation:

♦ Moving your eyes slowly right and left as you do this will help with spatial awareness.

TUNE IN (3 MIN)

Why:

When we massage the ears, we balance the energy in the whole body. This auricular exercise stimulates over 140 acupuncture points in the ear, creating a feeling of liveliness and alertness. It also enhances listening skills as well as focus and concentration.

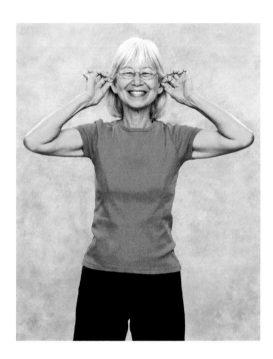

How:

◆ Pinch the tops of your ears.

◆ Use thumb and index fingers to massage and "unroll" the outer part of the ear.

◆ Pull ears gently out and back as you work down to the bottom lobe.

◆ Do this several times.

Variation:

◆ Cross your arms and massage the left ear with the right hand and the right ear with the left hand.

◆ Alternate squatting (inhale) and standing (exhale) as you stimulate ear lobes with crossed arms.

CROSS-CRAWL (10 MIN)

Why:

We discovered balance when we first learned to crawl. We perfected balance when we started to walk, then to run. Moving the left leg activates the right hemisphere of the brain. Moving the right arm activates the left hemisphere. Bringing the two together at the mid-line requires communication through a brain structure called the corpus callosum, a kind of neurological traffic cop. Right-left coordination governs our skills of locomotion, posture, and balance.

Whole-body coordination requires that we exercise bilateral skills. When the analytical left brain and the reflexive/rhythmic right brain are equally activated, any physical or mental experience is easier. This is why activities that make us cross the visual mid-line, practice whole-body coordination, and improve binocular vision will help us keep on moving and perceiving with balance.

Cross-Crawl is helpful in enhancing coordination and preventing falls as you get older. As you do the activity, imagine yourself power-walking with arms swinging, ice-skating rhythmically, or cross-country skiing with fluid grace.

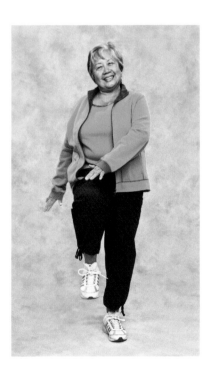

How:
BASIC CROSS-CRAWL (5 MIN)

- ◆ March in place, lifting the knees high.

- ◆ At the same time, reach across and touch the knee with the opposite hand or elbow. Right hand to left knee; left hand to right knee. Alternate and keep going.

- ◆ If you cannot lift your knees high, adapt the activity to your limitations. For example, step out in front, placing the foot on the floor and touching knee with opposite hand. Or do this sitting.

- ◆ You can do Cross-Crawl sitting, standing, moving, or lying down.

COGNITIVE CROSS-CRAWL (10 MIN)

◆ Close your eyes while doing the cross-crawl movement. This really causes the vestibular system— your mechanism of balance—to do its work!

◆ Open your eyes. Look around in all directions while doing cross-crawl movement.

◆ Walk, eyes slowly shifting to look in all directions. Vary your walking speed. Slow, then quick.

◆ Do the cross-crawl movement while counting backwards from one hundred by twos or by threes. This activity combines integrative movement with cognitive skill. You'll have to slow way down to do this one. Your partner checks for accuracy. If you don't have a partner, you'll have to check yourself for accuracy.

CROSS-CRAWL RAP (3–5 MIN)

(from Victoria Tennant)

◆ Do the Cross-Crawl while reciting the following "rap" in unison. Each line of the rap has four beats.

◆ Do the cross-mid-line action on beats two and four, alternating between right and left.

(hand to knee)
Cross tap, cross tap,
Cross the brain bridge with this rap.

(elbow to knee)
Elbow knee, elbow knee,
Learning can be fun for me.

(hand to heel either behind or in front of you)
Hand heel, hand heel,
I can change the way I feel.

(step forward and snap opposite fingers)
Cross snap, cross snap,
Use my whole brain with this rap.

INFINITY CROSS-CRAWL (2 MIN)

◆ Extend both arms forward and do "Lazy 8s" (see page 20). Draw the infinity sign with both hands, starting in the middle and moving up to the right or up to the left.

◆ As your hands circle to the right, lift the right knee. As your hands circle to the left, lift the left knee. Be aware of what is going on with your arms and what is going on with your legs. Notice the Cross-Crawl. Notice the Lazy 8 (infinity sign).

◆ Do this as you slowly turn your head to the right, and then to the left.

◆ Add a cognitive task.

You The Dancer (10-15 min)

Why:

Imagine that you are a dancer, and so do these activities with deliberate grace, balance, and coordination. You will be using the right and left sides of your body at the same time, integrating the right and left hemispheres of your brain. Successful integration improves all brain processes, including those for motor skills, physical coordination, and cognition.

There are five variations. Each one takes two to four minutes to perform. Repeat each dancer pose several times. You can do just one or else mix and vary them, creating a sequence that suits your physical abilities. Such a sequence can last from ten to fifteen minutes. Put on some lovely music.

How:

Side Leg-Raise Dancer

- ◆ Hold onto a chair if needed.
- ◆ Lift your right leg to the side about twelve inches or as far as is comfortable.
- ◆ At the same time, extend your right hand straight out in front of you.
- ◆ Drop your right hand and extend your left hand straight out in front of you.
- ◆ Keep your back and both legs straight.
- ◆ Repeat with left leg and left arm, and then left leg and right arm.
- ◆ Hold each dancer pose for several seconds. Increase holding time.

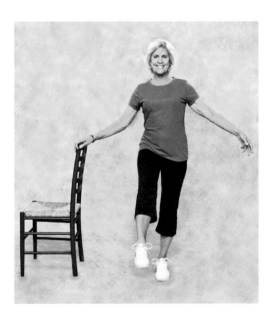

Forward Leg-Raise Dancer

- ◆ Hold onto a chair if needed.
- ◆ Lift your right leg out in front of you.
- ◆ Extend your right arm out to your side.
- ◆ Drop your right arm, and extend your left arm out to your side (see photo).
- ◆ Repeat with left leg and left arm, and then left leg and right arm.
- ◆ Hold each dancer pose for several seconds. Increase holding time.

FORWARD TOE-TOUCH DANCER

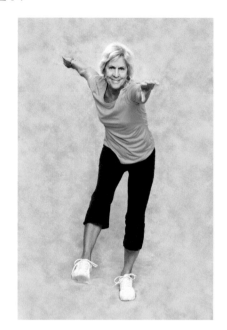

- Hold onto a chair if needed.

- Place your feet shoulder-width apart.

- Place your hands at your shoulders, palms forward.

- Simultaneously extend your right arm and your left foot forward.

- Point down with your left toes and touch the floor, or keep the toes a few inches off the floor (more difficult).

- Then repeat with left arm and right foot.

- Hold each dancer pose for several seconds. Increase holding time.

- Advanced: Do a "Charleston" move with one arm forward and one arm back as in the photo.

LEG-BACK DANCER

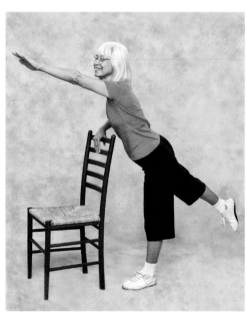

- Hold onto a chair if needed.

- Extend your left arm in front of you while you lift your left leg behind you (see photo). Hold several seconds.

- Bend the right leg until the left foot touches the floor, heel down. This is a typical runner's stretch. Hold several seconds.

- Repeat by extending your left arm forward and your right leg back. Bend the left leg until the right foot touches the floor, heel down. Hold several seconds.

- Repeat by extending your right arm forward and your right leg back. Bend the left leg until the right foot touches the floor, heel down. Hold several seconds.

- Repeat by extending your right arm forward and your left leg back. Bend the right leg until the left foot touches the floor, heel down. Hold several seconds.

- In each case, hold the position with your back foot off the floor and then hold the position with your heel down on the floor.

- Keep your back straight and your abs tight.

- Hold each dancer pose for several seconds. Increase holding time.

SIDE-LUNGE DANCER

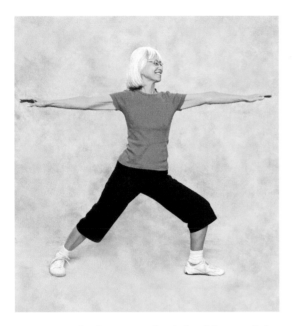

- ◆ Hold onto a chair if needed.

- ◆ Start with feet together.

- ◆ Step to the side with the left foot so that your feet are perpendicular.

- ◆ Bend the left knee as if lunging.

- ◆ Hold your arms out to your sides, shoulder height, as in the photo.

- ◆ Hold for several seconds.

- ◆ Return to neutral position, with feet together.

- ◆ Repeat the lunge to the right, with arms out to your sides.

- ◆ Repeat the lunge to the left with your right arm straight out in front.

- ◆ Repeat the lunge to the left with your left arm straight out in front.

- ◆ Repeat the lunge to the right with your left arm straight out in front.

- ◆ Repeat the lunge to the right with your right arm straight out in front.

- ◆ Hold each dancer pose several seconds. Increase holding time.

Advanced Variation:

- ◆ Really feel yourself being a dancer. Exaggerate.

- ◆ Alternate between any two of the five "You the Dancer" movements. For example, do one Side-Leg Dancer (side leg and arm front) and alternate that with one Forward-Leg Raise Dancer (forward leg and side arm). Repeat the alternating.

- ◆ Add a cognitive task, such as doing simple math problems or counting backwards, while doing the dancer poses.

BALLS

(adapted from Edvin Manniko, O.D.)

Tennis balls come into play for the activities on pages 32 through 38. It's easy to find tennis balls in most neighborhoods.

Tennis balls come into play for the activities on pages 32 through 38.

Why:

Ball exercises are great for practicing dynamic visual tracking, improving reaction time, and keeping you focused and alert. When our eyes gather information, they send twenty percent of it directly to the motor centers of the brain, bypassing the visual cortex. This information is critical for eye-body and eye-hand coordination—in other words, for "visual motor integration" (balance and movement). Faster than thought, the eyes lead and the muscles follow. The activities below are designed to sharpen those "follow the leader" skills. Remember to "keep your eye on the ball." For a real challenge, add a cognitive task while playing ball.

How:

SOLO ONE-BALL PLAY (15–20 MIN)

Ball Toss

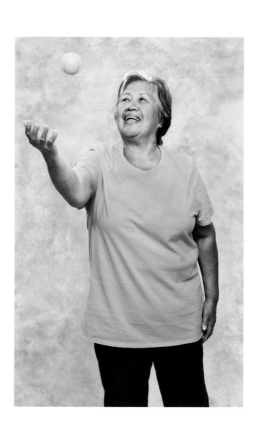

- ◆ While sitting, hold a tennis ball in your right hand. If sitting is too easy, start out standing.

- ◆ Toss the ball straight up. Keep your eyes on the ball.

- ◆ Catch it with your right hand.

- ◆ Shift hands. Toss and catch with the left hand.

- ◆ Strive for a juggling rhythm.

- ◆ Hold ball in the right hand, toss, and catch with the left.

- ◆ Hold ball in the left hand, toss, and catch with the right.

- ◆ Repeat this sequence while standing.

- ◆ Repeat while walking forward and backward.

- ◆ Repeat while reciting a poem.

- ◆ Vary the speed.

- ◆ Synchronize your tosses with a partner or a group.

Ball Bounce

- While sitting, hold the ball in your right hand. If sitting is too easy, start out standing.
- Bounce the ball and catch it with your right hand.
- Switch hands. Bounce and catch the ball with your left hand.
- Strive for a juggling rhythm.
- Bounce with the right hand and catch with the left.
- Bounce with the left hand and catch with the right.
- Repeat while standing.
- Repeat while walking forward and back.
- Vary the speed.

Alternate Ball Toss & Bounce

- Start with the right hand. Bounce, catch. Toss, catch.
- Now the left hand. Bounce, catch. Toss, catch.
- Mix up the tossing hand and the catching hand.
- Repeat while walking forward and back.
- Vary the speed.

Ball Toss with Clap

- Hold ball in right hand.
- Toss the ball in the air.
- Clap your hands.
- Catch the ball in your right hand.
- Repeat this with the left hand.
- Mix up the tossing and catching hands while clapping during each toss.
- Keep in rhythm while making patterns.
- Repeat while walking forward and back.
- Vary the speed.

Ball Bounce with Clap

- ◆ Hold ball in right hand.
- ◆ Bounce the ball.
- ◆ While it's bouncing, clap your hands.
- ◆ Catch the ball in your right hand.
- ◆ Repeat this with the left hand.
- ◆ Mix up the bouncing and catching hands while clapping during each bounce.
- ◆ Keep in rhythm while making patterns.
- ◆ Mix bouncing and tossing actions, continuing to clap every time the ball is in motion.
- ◆ Repeat these activities while walking forward and back.
- ◆ Vary the speed.

SOLO TWO-BALL PLAY   (15–20 MIN)

Why:

Double the balls means double the fun—and twice the benefits for balance, coordination, alertness, and visual motor integration.

How:

Double Ball Toss

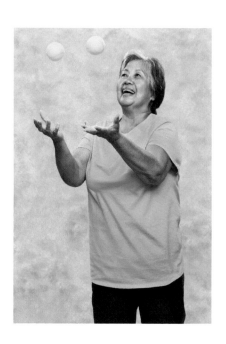

- ◆ Hold a tennis ball in each hand.
- ◆ Toss both balls up at the same time.
- ◆ Catch each ball in the hand that tossed it.
- ◆ Repeat while walking forward and back.

Double Ball Bounce

- ◆ Hold a tennis ball in each hand.
- ◆ Bounce both balls at the same time.
- ◆ Catch each ball in the hand that bounced it.
- ◆ Repeat while walking forward and back.

Alternate Double Ball Toss & Bounce

- ◆ Hold a tennis ball in each hand.
- ◆ Toss both balls up at the same time.
- ◆ Catch each ball in the hand that tossed it.
- ◆ Bounce both balls at the same time.
- ◆ Catch each ball in the hand that bounced it.
- ◆ Repeat while walking forward and back.
- ◆ Vary the speed. Keep in rhythm.

PARTNER ONE-BALL PLAY (15–30 MIN)

Why:

Working with a partner adds tremendously to the benefits of these activities. You have to be on your toes because you have to anticipate when your partner will move. Coordinated movements and fast reaction time indicate good brain processing ability, which is necessary for cognitive skills and balance. Follow the ball with your eyes. After some practice, try synchronizing your bounces and claps.

How:

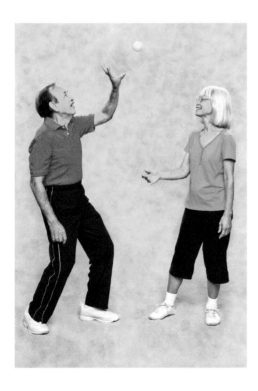

One-Ball Toss

- ◆ Hold ball in your right hand.
- ◆ Toss to partner.
- ◆ Partner catches ball with right hand, tosses it back.
- ◆ Catch with right hand.
- ◆ Repeat.
- ◆ Shift to left hands, tossing and catching.
- ◆ Find a rhythm.
- ◆ Toss with right hand, catch with left. Toss left, catch right.
- ◆ Mix it up. Tosser calls out which hand to catch with. Catcher calls out which hand to toss with.
- ◆ Repeat while slowly walking forward and back.

One-Ball Bounce

♦ Hold ball in your right hand.

♦ Bounce to partner.

♦ Partner catches ball with right hand, bounces it back.

♦ Catch with right hand.

♦ Shift to left hands, bouncing and catching.

♦ Mix it up, as before. Call out to each other. Find a rhythm.

♦ Do this while walking.

Alternate One-Ball Toss & Bounce

♦ Following the same progression, this time alternate between tosses and bounces.

♦ Right hands.

♦ Left hands.

♦ Mix it up.

♦ Find a rhythm.

♦ Walk forward and back.

One-Ball Toss with Clap

♦ Repeat One-Ball Toss. This time, add partner claps every time the ball is mid-toss.

One-Ball Bounce with Clap

♦ Repeat One-Ball Bounce. This time, add partner claps every time the ball is mid-bounce.

Alternate One-Ball Toss with Clap & One-Ball Bounce with Clap

♦ Put it all together.

♦ Start with right-to-right toss with claps. Play catch.

♦ Do right-to-right bounce with claps.

♦ Shift to left-to-left toss with claps, then left-to-left bounce with claps.

♦ Mix it up, calling out to each other.

♦ Repeat while walking forward and back.

♦ Stay focused.

Foot Catch

- Stand facing a partner. If standing is difficult, do this seated.
- Trap a ball under your right foot.
- Roll the ball with your foot toward the partner.
- Partner traps the ball with the right foot.
- Switch to left foot. Roll and "catch" with left feet.
- Mix it up, partners calling which foot to catch with.
- Alternate feet while counting backwards from one hundred by twos or threes.
- Have a conversation while doing the foot-rolling.
- Add another ball.

PARTNER TWO-BALL PLAY

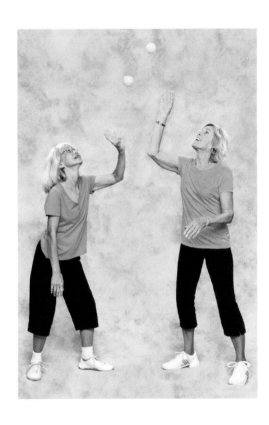

Double Ball Toss and Catch

- Each partner holds a ball.
- Toss ball to partner as partner tosses ball to you.
- Partners catch both balls at the same time.
- Vary the height by tossing and catching at different levels (low, medium, high).
- Increase the challenge by walking forward and back while playing catch with two balls. Or take turns counting backwards from one hundred by twos or by threes. Or have a conversation while playing catch in this way.

Double Ball Bounce and Catch

- As the previous, but this time you and your partner are bouncing, not tossing.

Alternate Double Ball Toss & Double Ball Bounce and Catch

◆ Alternate between two-ball tossing and two-ball bouncing while continuing to play catch in this fashion.

PARTNER FOUR-BALL PLAY

Four-Ball Toss and Catch

◆ Each partner holds a ball in each hand.

◆ Partners toss and catch simultaneously.

Four-Ball Bounce and Catch

◆ Each partner holds a ball in each hand.

◆ Partners bounce and catch simultaneously.

Alternate Four-Ball Toss & Four-Ball Bounce and Catch

◆ Each partner holds a ball in each hand.

◆ Partners toss and catch simultaneously alternating with a bounce and catch simultaneously.

GROUP BALL PLAY

Twist & Reach

◆ Four to six people stand back to back in a circle.

◆ Two people start passing balls around the circle.

◆ Twist as you pass a ball.

◆ Repeat this several times, twisting and passing.

◆ Reverse the direction.

◆ Vary the heights (low, medium, high).

◆ Go slowly at first, then speed up.

◆ Add more balls.

Foot Catch

◆ See Partner One-Ball Play for instructions, but do in a group of four to six.

BEANBAGS

Why:

Who would have thought that beanbags could be the secret to a better life? They are essential for the activities on pages 39 through 41. You can make your own beanbags at home, or you can easily find them in a neighborhood store. These activities are similar to the ball play of the previous section, but beanbags are easier to toss and catch. Of course, they're impossible to bounce. In fact, try to keep them off the floor so that they stay clean.

How:

SOLO ONE-BEANBAG PLAY (5–10 MIN)

Each exercise takes 2–3 minutes.

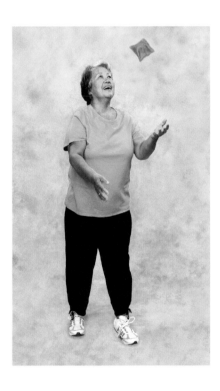

One-Beanbag Toss

◆ Toss and catch with the right hand.

◆ Toss and catch with the left hand.

◆ Toss back and forth between hands.

◆ Find a rhythm.

◆ Repeat while walking forwards and back.

◆ Variation: Count backwards from one hundred by twos or threes.

One-Beanbag Toss with Clap

◆ Repeat One-Beanbag Toss. This time, clap every time the beanbag is aloft.

SOLO TWO-BEANBAG PLAY

(5–10 MIN)

Double Beanbag Toss

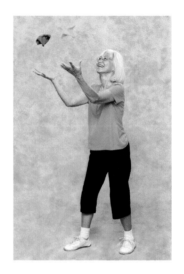

- ◆ Hold a beanbag in each hand.
- ◆ Toss both beanbags in the air simultaneously and catch each one with the hand that tossed it.
- ◆ Repeat while walking and counting.

PARTNER ONE-BEANBAG PLAY

(10–15 MIN)

Each of these takes approximately 3–5 minutes.

One-Beanbag Catch

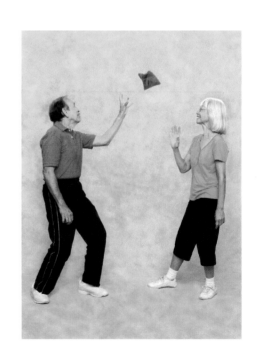

- ◆ Stand with a partner ready to play catch, a beanbag in your right hand.
- ◆ Toss the beanbag so that your partner catches it in the right hand.
- ◆ Shift to the left hand, partner catching with the left hand.
- ◆ Shift to cross-handed tossing, right-to-left and left-to-right. Partners call out which hand to toss with, which to catch with.
- ◆ Find a juggling rhythm.
- ◆ Repeat while walking and counting. One partner checks the other for accuracy.

One-Beanbag Catch with Clap

- ◆ Do the previous. But this time the partners clap together every time the beanbag gets tossed.

PARTNER TWO-BEANBAG PLAY (10–15 MIN)

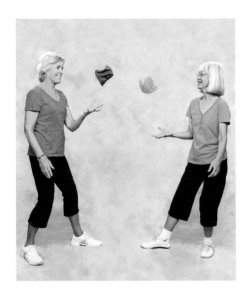

Double Beanbag Catch

◆ Stand facing partner.

◆ Each partner has a beanbag.

◆ Play catch simultaneously, each tossing a beanbag. Partners catch beanbags at the same time.

◆ Vary height by catching at different levels (low, medium, high).

◆ Repeat while walking slowly forward and back.

◆ Repeat while taking turns counting or while having a conversation.

Four Beanbag Catch

◆ Each partner holds a beanbag in each hand.

◆ Partners toss and catch simultaneously

◆ Same variations as above.

GROUP BEANBAG PLAY (5–10 MIN)

Twist & Reach

◆ Four to six people stand back to back in a circle.

◆ Two people start passing beanbags around the circle.

◆ Twist as you pass a beanbag.

◆ Repeat this several times, twisting and passing.

◆ Reverse the direction.

◆ Vary the heights (low, medium, high).

◆ Go slowly at first, then speed up.

◆ Pass overhead, then through the legs.

◆ Add more beanbags.

CONFIDENCE WALK

Why:

Walking is such an important part of our everyday lives. You can actually practice walking with balance. Move With Balance!

This might take twenty to thirty minutes for the full sequence. You can always mix and match.

CONFIDENCE WALK PRE- AND POST-TEST

♦ You may want to pre- and post-test the Confidence Walk sequence, but it isn't necessary. Check your walk before and after you do the movements.

♦ Walk forward at your normal speed. Notice how you walk. How do you feel?

♦ Notice posture, breathing, head position. Where are your eyes? Notice how your feet touch the floor. Is your weight evenly distributed?

How:

BALANCE WALK

♦ Tape an eight-foot strip of masking tape or string to the floor. Walk on the tape. (You can also do this without the tape or string.)

♦ Stand up with good posture. Hold a few seconds. Breathe.

♦ Keep your head and eyes up if you can. Choose a spot ahead of you and focus on it to keep steady as you walk.

♦ Move slowly and carefully, forward and then backwards.

♦ As your foot touches the ground, the momentum is heel-to-toe when walking forward and toe-to-heel walking backwards.

♦ Use the arm of a partner if you need to, but notice what you are doing.

♦ Advanced Variation: Vary the length of your gait. Vary speed.

♦ More advanced: As you walk, lift your back leg. Pause for a second before stepping forward. Alternate the paused leg.

♦ Add a cognitive task, like counting or reciting a poem.

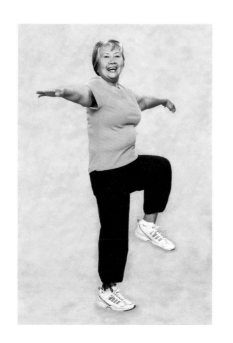

High-Step Walk

- Walk the line. This time, exaggerate by bringing each leg up very high.
- Vary by pausing between high steps.
- Slowly turn head right and left as you walk.
- Walk forward and backward.

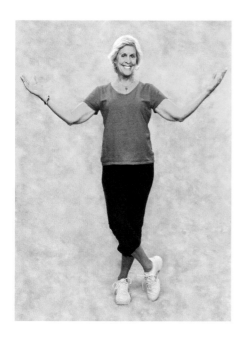

Side-Step Walk

- Walk sidestepping. Bring the right foot across the left and step down three to five inches away from the left foot. Ankles are crossed. The closer the feet, the harder it is to balance.
- Alternate crossing the foot in front and then behind the other foot as you move along. Repeat several times.
- Then bring the left foot across three to five inches next to the right foot. Repeat several times.
- Practice walking this way. Head up, good posture.
- Advanced variation: place feet closer together when you cross ankles.

TIGHTROPE WALK

- ◆ Place the heel of one foot directly in front of the toe of the other foot, as if you are beginning to walk on a tightrope.

- ◆ Put your arms out to the side like a tightrope walker.

- ◆ Choose a spot ahead of you and focus on it with your eyes. This will help to keep you steady as you walk.

- ◆ Stand still for a count of ten.

- ◆ Keep going like this, stepping and stopping, until you have reached the end of the tape.

- ◆ Gradually increase the ten-count to thirty seconds.

- ◆ Do without stopping and pausing.

- ◆ Walk backwards.

- ◆ If necessary, place your feet wider apart.

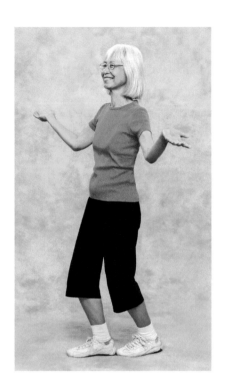

INFINITY WALK

- ◆ Walk the infinity pattern on the floor. (See Lazy 8s, page 20.)

WALK WITH HEAD-TURNS

- ◆ Walk forward normally.

- ◆ As you walk, turn your head to the left and continue to walk.

- ◆ Then turn your head to the right and continue.

- ◆ Slowly walk backwards as you turn your head left and then right.

- ◆ The head turns are as if you are turning your head to look at something.

- ◆ Change the movement of your head. Move it up and down as if nodding.

- ◆ Walk forward and back at various speeds.

- ◆ Lengthen your gait. Shorten it.

- ◆ Advanced: Read words or letters from the Vision Card in Appendix B as you turn your head.

FOCUS ON YOUR FEET

Why:

By training the body to pay attention to the feet and by strengthening the muscles used in standing, these activities improve your sense of balance and prevent falls. If necessary, hang onto a chair while you do these.

How:

HEEL LIFTS (2 MIN)

- ◆ Stand up straight.
- ◆ Slowly rise up on your tiptoes.
- ◆ Hold for three counts.
- ◆ Lower your heels back to the floor.
- ◆ Once this is easy, do one foot at a time.

TOE LIFTS (2 MIN)

- ◆ Stand up straight.
- ◆ Lift your toes off the floor.
- ◆ Don't let your hips move backwards.
- ◆ Hold for three counts.
- ◆ Lower your toes back to the floor.
- ◆ Advanced Variation: roll through the foot, heel to toe, toe to heel.

ONE-FOOT CONVERSATION (3 MIN)

- ◆ Work with a partner.
- ◆ Stand on one foot.
- ◆ While doing that, have a conversation with your partner.
- ◆ When you start to feel wobbly, switch to the other foot.
- ◆ Variation: While standing on one foot, reach across to your partner and lightly touch opposite hands.

TOES AND EYES

Why:

The next two activities connect with important energy points in the body. One goes from above the upper lip to the tailbone. The other goes from below the lower lip to navel. These two activities help to focus concentration, improve balance, and ground you solidly in your body.

How:

TOES AND EYES I (3 MIN)

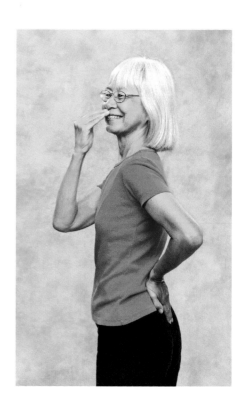

- ◆ Put your fingers on the space above your upper lip and the fingers of your other hand on your lower spine (your sacrum).

- ◆ Rise up on your toes. Then come back down fully. Move through your feet, fully feeling the bottoms of your feet as you move through them. Continue rising and returning.

- ◆ Add simultaneous moving of your eyes up and down, tracking a vertical plane.

- ◆ Add the breath. Breathe in with eyes up and rising up on your toes. Breathe out with eyes down and the energy moving down through your feet, heels down.

- ◆ Coordinate this pattern rhythmically.

- ◆ Shift hands, putting the opposite fingers on your lower spine and above your upper lip.

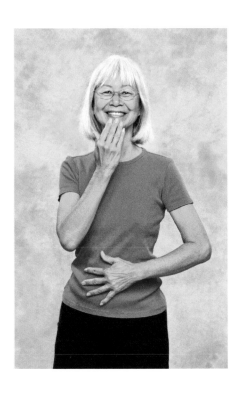

TOES AND EYES II (3 MIN)

- ◆ Put your fingers under your lower lip and the fingers of your other hand on your navel.

- ◆ Rise up on your toes. Then come back down fully. Move through your feet, fully feeling the bottoms of your feet as you move through them. Continue rising and returning.

- ◆ Add simultaneous moving of your eyes up and down, tracking a vertical plane.

- ◆ Add the breath. Breathe in with eyes up and rising up on your toes. Breathe out with eyes down and the energy moving down through your feet, heels down.

- ◆ Coordinate this pattern rhythmically.

- ◆ Shift hands, putting the opposite fingers on your navel and under your lower lip.

GAIT POINTS (5 MIN)

(from Touch for Health)

Why:

This exercise helps the normal coordination of muscles used in walking.

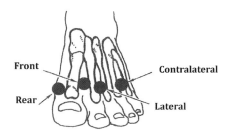

How:

- ◆ Firmly massage appropriate gait points on both feet.

- ◆ These are located at the top of the joining of toes and foot. See diagram.

- ◆ Place your fingers on the bottom of the foot as your thumb stimulates each point.

KICK BALL CHANGE (3 MIN)

Why:

Shifting your weight from the left to the right foot forces you to balance on one foot. By having to keep in rhythm, you are forced to process information quickly and accurately. Poor brain timing and slow reaction time are improved. Kick Ball Change is a jazz dance step that you can do alone or in a group.

How:

- ◆ Put on some jazzy music.
- ◆ Give yourself room to move.
- ◆ Kick with the right foot, step on the ball of the right foot, then shift your weight to the left foot.
- ◆ Repeat several times.
- ◆ Kick with the left foot, step on the ball of the left foot, then change to right foot.
- ◆ Repeat several times.
- ◆ Now alternate between right and left. Kick right, step right, change to left; kick left, step left, change to right. Keep in the rhythm. Dance away.

THE CAT JUMP (3 MIN)

Why:

This activity is to practice catching yourself should you ever fall. The muscle memory of this movement is etched in your body.

How:

- ◆ Bend your knees in a squat.
- ◆ Jump a little off the ground with both feet.
- ◆ Land softly, like a cat, not jarring your body.
- ◆ Repeat several times until you are comfortable doing it.

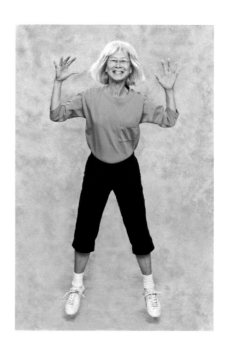

STRENGTHEN YOUR LEGS

 Why:

Nothing could be more important in fall-prevention than good lower-body strength. These activities will also make it easier for you to climb stairs and get in and out of a car. Do the following activities while holding onto the back of a chair. Start with two hands on the chair. As you gain strength, use just one hand, then one finger, and then no hands. Each sequence takes about 5-7 minutes.

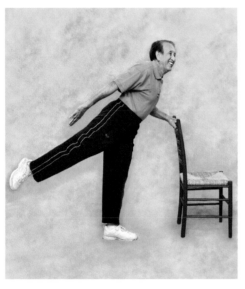

How:

BACK-LEG RAISE (3 MIN)

- ◆ Stand behind a sturdy chair with feet slightly apart.
- ◆ Do the activity four times in this sequence with each leg: Two hands, one hand, one finger, no hands.
- ◆ Slowly lift one leg straight back without bending your knee or pointing your toes.
- ◆ Do your best not to lean forward. The leg you are standing on should be slightly bent.
- ◆ Hold this position. Increase the holding time.
- ◆ Slowly lower your leg.

- ◆ Repeat five to ten times with each hand position.
- ◆ Shift to the other leg and repeat five to ten times with each hand position.
- ◆ Advanced: Rest and repeat the activity.

SIDE-LEG RAISE (3 MIN)

- ◆ Stand behind a sturdy chair with feet slightly apart.
- ◆ Do the activity four times in this sequence with each leg: Two hands, one hand, one finger, no hands.
- ◆ Slowly lift one leg out to the side.
- ◆ Keep your back straight and your toes facing forward. The leg you are standing on should be slightly bent.
- ◆ Hold this position. Increase the holding time.
- ◆ Slowly lower your leg.
- ◆ Repeat five to ten times with each hand position.
- ◆ Shift to the other leg and repeat five to ten times with each hand position.
- ◆ Advanced: Rest and repeat the activity.

KNEE CURL (3 MIN)

- ◆ Stand behind a sturdy chair, feet slightly apart.

- ◆ Do the activity four times in this sequence with each leg: Two hands, one hand, one finger, no hands.

- ◆ Lift one leg straight back, bending your knee.

- ◆ Slowly bring your heel up toward your buttocks as far as possible.

- ◆ Bend only from your knee, and keep your hips still. The leg you are standing on should be slightly bent.

- ◆ Hold this position. Increase the holding time.

- ◆ Slowly lower your foot to the floor.

- ◆ Repeat five to ten times with each hand position.

- ◆ Shift to the other leg and repeat five to ten times with each hand position.

- ◆ Advanced: Rest and repeat the activity.

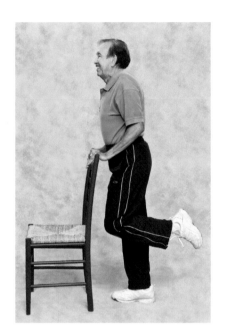

CHAIR STAND (3 MIN)

- ◆ Sit toward the front of a sturdy, armless chair with feet flat on floor, shoulder-width apart.

- ◆ Cross your hands over your chest.

- ◆ Keep your back and shoulders straight throughout this activity.

- ◆ As you slowly stand, extend your arms so that they are parallel to the floor.

- ◆ Slowly sit down again.

- ◆ Repeat this activity five to ten times.

- ◆ Advanced: Rest and repeat the activity.

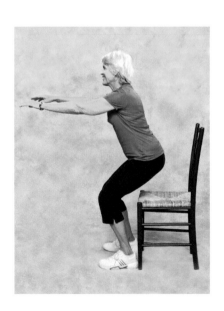

CHILDHOOD GAMES

Why:

Smooth, coordinated movements are the result of precise timing and good integration between the two sides of the brain. These sensory integration activities trigger the timing processes in the brain. To do them, you need to move both sides of your body rhythmically, with precise movements, while singing or playing a game. Rhymes and songs are excellent focusing devices, especially when performed with matching movements. There's a reason why these silly songs have stood the test of time.

"Row Your Boat" and the "Hokey Pokey" are a lot of fun to perform in groups, ranging from as few as four or five people to as many as the room can hold. Working in a group motivates individuals and removes some of the tedium of repetitive activities.

"Rock Paper Scissors (Cock Hen Chick)" is a variation of a game most of us played as children. It is done with a partner.

How:

HOKEY POKEY (5 MIN)

♦ Stand in a circle with a group. Leave enough room so that people don't bump into one another.
♦ Sing "The Hokey Pokey Song."
♦ While singing, do the actions the song demands.

The Hokey Pokey Song:

You put your right foot in.

You put your right foot out.

You put your right foot in

And you shake it all about.

You do the Hokey Pokey

And you turn yourself around—

That's what it's all about. (two claps)

Words and music by Larry LaPrise

The sequence:

♦ right foot
♦ left foot
♦ right hand
♦ left hand
♦ right shoulder
♦ left shoulder
♦ right hip
♦ left hip
♦ whole self

ROW YOUR BOAT (7–10 MIN)

(from Jon Bredal)

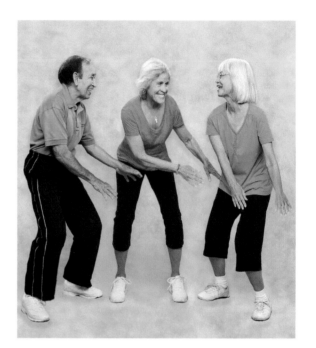

- Sit or stand in a circle with shoulders almost touching. Partners can face each other. Each time you add a head movement, it becomes more challenging.

- Sing "Row Your Boat" with the following hand gestures:

    row, row, — move hands to the left with two beats.

    row your boat — tap your thighs with two beats.

    gently down the — move hands to the right with two beats.

    stream — tap your thighs with two beats.

- Keep singing, in addition to the arms, add head movements that go opposite the hand movements. When your hands move left, look to the right. When your hands move right, look to the left.

- Do this for a while until you "get it."

- Keep singing, this time adding a head movement up and a head movement down matching the tapping of the thighs. Like so:

    row, row, — hands left two beats, look right.

    row your boat — tap thighs two beats, look up.

    gently down the —hands right two beats, look left.

    stream —tap thighs two beats, look down.

- Do this for a while until you "get it."

- Laughing is always okay.

Rock Paper Scissors (Cock Hen Chick) (7–10 min)

(from Conrad Ho and Amy Choi)

Why:

In this activity participants must do several things at the same time, and each thing must be done with appropriate timing. Success requires high concentration in the moment, and it requires flawless coordination among verbal cues, hand gestures, brain decisions, and sequencing of actions.

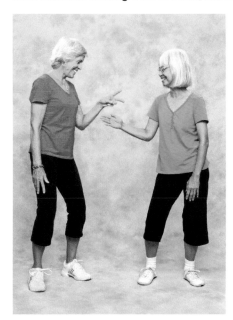

These skills are exactly what you need for effective verbal communication and sensory integration. Winning is determined not only by the "rock paper scissors" outcome but also by indicating the outcome. Every act in the process is important as you do the right thing at the right time. More advanced players may accelerate the pace to confuse their opponents.

How:

◆ Face a partner, sitting or standing.

◆ With a one-two rhythm partners clap, clap, then thrust out a hand in the shape of either "rock" (a fist), "paper" (flat hand palm down), or "scissors" (index and long fingers extended in V shape).

◆ Winning is determined this way: rock breaks scissors, paper covers rock, scissors cuts paper.

◆ Without hesitation, repeat the pattern of clap, clap, thrust. This time, show the outcome of the contest using hand gestures: "cock" (the winner puts hand on head like a cock's comb), "hen" (in a tie, both partners make chicken wings and waggle their elbows), or "chick" (the loser puts hand on tailbone to suggest tail feathers).

◆ Immediately repeat the game.

◆ Keep in rhythm.

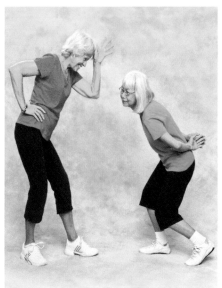

KNEE OVER BALL O'LEARY (5–10 MIN)

Why:

Adding a schoolyard-style counting chant to a ball-bounce activity brings auditory and rhythmic elements to bear. As simple as this activity is, it exercises eye-brain-motor responses in many ways at once.

The chant has four lines. Each line has four counts. This activity asks you to bounce the ball on every count, also add a knee movement on the fourth count of every line when you chant the word "O'Leary."

One, two, three, O'Leary.

Four, five, six, O'Leary.

Seven, eight, nine, O'Leary.

Ten, O'Leary, say "whooo, hooo, hooo."

How:

◆ Place a tennis ball in your right hand.

◆ Each time you say a number, you bounce the ball.

◆ Each time you say "O'Leary," you move your right leg to the right over the ball.

◆ Repeat, holding the ball in your left hand and moving the left leg to the left over the ball.

Advanced Variations:

◆ Alternate right hand and left hand, right knee and left knee.

◆ Repeat the whole activity moving your knee inward, toward the center of your body.

SENSORY INTEGRATION

(from Bobbie Dirks, O.D.)

Activity Cards for the following movements are in Appendix B and on the website www.MoveWithBalance.org. You can laminate the cards, put the cards in plastic sheet protectors or use them as is. You might want to pick up the cards after each session.

Why:

Balance movements that integrate the visual, auditory, kinesthetic, tactile, and vestibular senses help to reduce injuries and improve performance. Neural capability and efficiency increases. Timing improves, vision improves, sense of balance improves, mental processing improves, and reaction time improves.

These movements allow us to practice this sensory motor integration. We can use them to challenge ourselves as we see, say, hear, touch, and move all at the same time.

How:

CLOCK FACE (7–15 MIN)

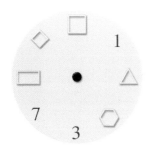

- ◆ Work with a partner. As you do the movement, have your partner check to see that you've given the right answers.

- ◆ If you do this movement alone, you'll have to check yourself, of course.

- ◆ Create a pattern by going around the clock face saying and touching what is in the place of the numbers on a clock.

- ◆ Example: start in the twelve o'clock position with the square. Touch the square on the clock and say *"square."* Then touch your nose and say *"nose."* Then touch the dot in the center of the clock and say *"dot."* Then touch your right ear and say *"ear."* That is the pattern—touch and say *"Square, nose, dot, ear"* using your right hand and right ear.

- ◆ Next, move to the numeral 1 in the one o'clock position and say *"one."* Then repeat the pattern: *"one, nose, dot, ear."*

- ◆ Touch the triangle in the next position. Say *"triangle, nose, dot, ear."*

- ◆ Do each pattern until you "get it" and then move to a new pattern.

- ◆ Notice that so far you have used only your right hand and right ear.

- ◆ Say the same pattern, but change the pattern by using the left hand and touching the left ear.

- ◆ Change to left hand and right ear. Continue to change the pattern as many times as you like.

- ◆ Go counterclockwise instead of clockwise.

- ◆ Keep a rhythm as you go around the clock. Rhythm is more important than speed.

- ◆ Advanced variation: alternate hands or ears every other time.

- ◆ When you're finished, switch roles and help your partner do the movements.

SLAP TAP (7–15 MIN)

- Do this sitting or standing.

- Work with a partner. As you do the activity, have your partner check to see that you've given the right answers.

- If you do this activity alone, you'll have to check yourself, of course.

- Look at the Slap Tap sheet. See the vertical line with the letter R or L either on the right or left side of the vertical line.

- The letters indicate which hand to use.

- The position of the letter on either side of the vertical line indicates which of your knees that hand is supposed to slap. Imagine that the vertical line is the center of your body.

  So:

    - If the letter R is on the right side of the vertical line, then slap your right knee with your right hand.

    - If the letter L is on the right side of the vertical line, then slap your right knee with your left hand.

    - If the letter R is on the left side of the vertical line, slap your left knee with your right hand.

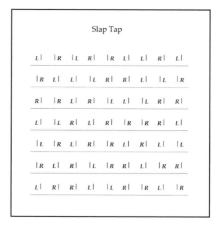

    - If the letter L is on the left side of the vertical line, slap your left knee with your left hand.

- "Read" the symbols on the Slap Tap one line, two lines, or the whole chart.

- Try to establish a rhythm. Rhythm is more important than speed.

- When you're finished, switch roles and help your partner do the activities.

- Advanced variation: Step forward with the same foot as the hand you are using.

ARROWS (15–20 MIN FOR COMPLETE SEQUENCE)

- Face a partner. While you do the activity, have your partner hold the arrow chart and check to see if you've given the correct answers.

- If you do this activity alone, you'll have to check yourself, of course.

- Look at the arrow chart and call out the direction indicated by the arrow. (Up, down, left, or right.) Then thrust your arms in that direction. In other words, say and do what the arrow indicates.

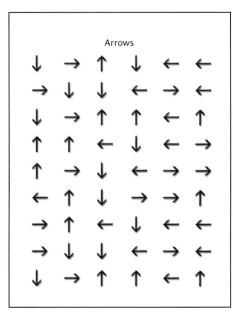

- "Read" the Arrow Chart, one line, two lines, or the whole chart.

- Next look at the arrow chart and call out the direction opposite the arrow. Thrust your hands in the direction opposite the arrow. In other words, say and do the opposite of what the arrow indicates. "Read" several lines.

- Next look at the Arrow Chart and call out the direction indicated by the arrow. But thrust your arms in the opposite direction. In other words, say what the arrow indicates but do the opposite. Read several lines.

- Next look at the arrow chart and call out the direction opposite the arrow. But thrust your arms in the direction indicated by the arrow. In other words, say the opposite of what the arrow indicates but do what it indicates. Read several lines.

- When you're finished, switch roles and help your partner do the activities.

- Advanced Variation: In addition to moving your arms, you can step right, left, forward for up, and backwards for down to match the arrow's direction or opposite the arrow's direction.

VISION AND BALANCE

Why:

The vestibular system (our balance) works with the visual system to detect head and body motion as well as eye movement. Improving the visual system can significantly boost performance by improving response time, vision-body coordination, balance, and confidence. As you do the next two movements, read the large letters/words on the Vision Card. See Appendix B or www.MoveWithBalance.org website to access the Vision Card. Fold the paper in half.

How:

VISION CARD BALANCE: HEAD MOVING (7–10 MIN)

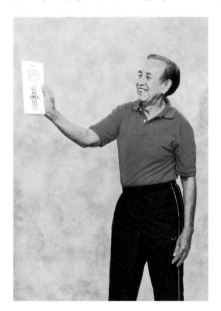

◆ Hold the Vision Card still while you focus on the biggest letters.

◆ Stand, feet shoulder width apart.

◆ Move your head from side to side while continuing to keep the letters in clear focus.

◆ Move your head up and down, like nodding, while you keep the letters in focus.

◆ Move your head diagonally, both ways, while focusing on the letters.

◆ Repeat with feet together, then with one foot in front of the other. This is a lot more difficult.

VISION CARD BALANCE: HEAD STILL (7–10 MIN)

◆ Hold the Vision Card as before.

◆ Hold your head still.

◆ Stand, feet shoulder width apart.

◆ Move the card from side to side while you continue to keep the letters in clear focus.

◆ Move the card up and down while you stay focused on the letters.

◆ Move the card diagonally, both ways, while focusing on the letters.

◆ Repeat with feet together, then with one foot in front of the other.

Sharpen Your Vision with Fusion

Why:

When the brain takes information from both eyes and merges that into a single image, we call that "fusion." Fusion gives us depth perception, the ability to see three-dimensionally. Usually we do it unconsciously. But when we become conscious of fusion, we can enhance or improve it, or we can become aware that it's not happening. People without fusion might not even know it because the brain compensates. But such compensation is wasted energy. The Move With Balance® movements help us use the brain/visual system as it was designed. They improve fusion and give us an exciting increase in clarity and depth perception.

Controlling how we use and aim our eyes together is an important skill.

There are two basic ways to aim or "team" our eyes:

1) Convergence: turning the eyes inward to maintain single vision for objects up close, similar to looking "cross-eyed."

2) Divergence: turning the eyes outward to maintain a single image for objects far away, apparently aiming straight ahead.

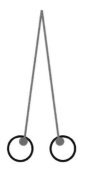
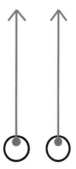

Vision Card for Pre-and Post-Testing (3 min)

(from Janet Goodrich)

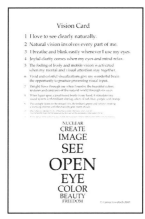

Use the Vision Card to pre- and post-check any changes in your sense of vision. The Vision Card lists eleven sentences from larger to smaller print. Hold the card at your normal reading distance. What is the smallest line you can read on the pre-test? After doing the activities, check again. What's the smallest line you can read on the post-test?

You do not have to use the Vision Card every time you do the fusion activities. But it is fun to notice changes and improvement. Be sure to hold the card in the same place for pre- and post-tests. Experiment with and without your glasses.

THUMB FUSION (10 MIN)

- ◆ Hold one thumb about eight inches in front of your nose.

- ◆ Look at an object in the distance. Your thumb will appear to have doubled. It's as if you are looking through your thumb or past your thumb at the object in the distance.

- ◆ This time, focus on your thumb. Look directly at your thumb. What is in the distance doubles.

- ◆ Alternate looking at thumb then looking at the object in the distance—"thumb, distant object, thumb, distant object." "Converge, diverge, converge, diverge." Keep noticing that what you look at is single and what you are not looking at is double.

- ◆ Gradually vary the distance the thumb is from your nose, bringing it closer or farther.

- ◆ Vary the speed.

- ◆ Remember to blink and breathe.

- ◆ Do sitting at first, then shift to standing, then to moving.

- ◆ If you have trouble seeing the two thumbs, start by looking at something in the distance. Then slowly bring your thumb into view, as though it is passing along the tip of your nose. It may take a while for the double images to "come in" because you may be in the habit of suppressing the vision in one eye. Practice will allow it to work. You cannot make this happen. Relax and breathe, and it will suddenly "pop in" or seem to appear. When that happens, your two eyes are working together.

EE FUSION (10 MIN)

The EE Fusion activity is more advanced than Thumb Fusion. Having your two eyes work together means that your two brain hemispheres are working together and that you have good depth perception. As we get older, we lose the ability to converge and diverge quickly. This is what we are practicing.

E   E

- ◆ Work with the EE on a piece of paper approximately 2.5x4 inches. (You can copy EE from Appendix B or print it off the website www.MoveWithBalance.org.)

- ◆ Hold the EE eight inches in front of you as you did with the thumb.

- ◆ Focus your vision on some object in the distance. Notice that the EE card now seems to say EEE (similar to how you saw two thumbs). Now you see three E's.

- ◆ Look at a point in front of the EE you are holding and you will notice EEE.

- ◆ Alternate looking "past EE, in front of EE, past EE in front of EE," diverge, converge, diverge, converge, always being aware of the three EEE. The brain is fusing the two images into a third, three-dimensional image.

- ◆ Do sitting at first, then shift to standing, then to moving.

- ◆ Be sure to breathe and relax. You cannot force this. The image just "pops in" or seems to appear.

- ◆ Move the EE closer than eight inches. You will really feel your eye muscles work.

- ◆ Rest with Palming, page 67.

INNER-TUBE FUSION (10–15 MIN)

(from Edward Friedman, O.D.)

♦ Work with the Inner-Tube card. You can copy it from Appendix B or print it off the website www.MoveWithBalance.org. Cut out on the dotted lines.

♦ Experiment first without glasses, then with glasses.

♦ As you practice looking first in front of (convergence) and then past (divergence) the inner tubes, you will see a third fused image in the middle. This new image will be three-dimensional, and it will read "FUSE CLEAR."

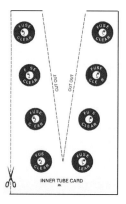

Convergence

♦ Place the white side of the folded Vision Card behind the inner tubes where you cut out the "V".

♦ Hold the Inner Tube Card eight inches from your nose.

♦ Look at a point in front of the inner tubes.

♦ Imagine a line connecting the tip of your nose to a point midway between the bottom circles. You may use your finger to guide you to this point.

♦ Begin at the bottom with the inner tubes that are closest together. You should now see that the two original inner tubes have fused into three. You may first see four, then three. Three is what you want to see.

♦ The center (third) image should be a fully fused image of the two originals. Notice that this third image is three-dimensional.

♦ Try to read the letters "FUSE CLEAR" on the fused image.

♦ Hold the fully fused image for the count of five.

♦ Repeat this routine for each inner tube pair, starting at the bottom.

Divergence

◆ Remove the folded Vision Card. Notice the "V".

◆ Select an object about fifteen feet away and look at it.

◆ Hold the Inner Tube Card about eight inches from your eyes.

◆ Fix your gaze through the "V" opening in the card, gazing at the distant object.

◆ Read "FUSE CLEAR" on the third image.

◆ If you see four circles, bring the two inner tubes closer together by bending the paper until you see three images, and then gradually move them apart. Three is what you want to see.

◆ You will feel your eyes trying to hold the fused image.

◆ Hold the fully fused image for the count of five.

Alternating Divergence and Convergence

◆ Alternate looking past (or through) the inner tubes with looking in front of the inner tubes— "past, in front of, past, in front of," always being aware of the three inner tubes of the fused image.

◆ Vary the distance of the card from your eyes.

◆ Hold the third image for a count of five, then for a count of ten.

◆ Do this with each set of inner tubes, starting at the bottom.

◆ The goal is to see the middle inner tube as a fused, three-dimensional image.

◆ Do sitting at first, then shift to standing, then to moving.

◆ Breathe and relax.

◆ Do Palming on page 67 to relax your eyes and give the brain a chance to absorb the movement.

◆ You may want to post-test yourself using the Vision Card after doing all the fusion activities.

INTEGRATION TIME: REST AND RELAX

You need "downtime" for your brain/body to integrate and absorb all the benefits of the Move With Balance® activities. Take integration time by resting and relaxing between and after activities.

CONNECT THE CIRCUITS (5 MIN)

(from Dr. Wayne Cook)

Why:

Wayne Cook, an expert in electromagnetic energy, created the following activity as a way to counter the effects of electromagnetic pollution—the result of sitting in front of a computer, television, or any other appliance that generates electromagnetic fields. His extensive research found that this posture has a harmonizing effect on the mind and body. We call it "Connect the Circuits."

This activity creates a whole-body figure-eight, balancing the energy in three dimensions. Do this whenever you experience feelings of anxiety, worry, or frustration. Be sure to do both parts and notice what happens as your concerns and anxieties melt. Notice the increased sensation of centeredness, clarity, and calm, comfort, balance, and coordination. "Connect the Circuits" encourages relaxation and integration time between activities. It connects the brain and body.

How:

Part One:

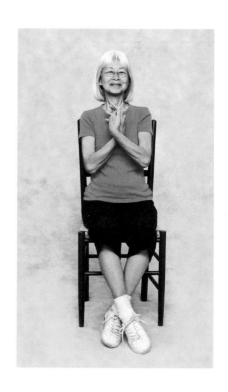

◆ While seated, cross one ankle over the other. Try it both ways until you find the combination that feels most comfortable and creates the greatest relaxation.

◆ Extend your arms, touching the backs of the hands together.

◆ Cross one hand over the other at the wrist, bringing the palms of the hands together thumbs down.

◆ With your fingers clasped together, move your hands up and through your arms, resting them comfortably on your heart with elbows at your sides.

◆ Breathe deeply and comfortably. Or you may want to touch the tongue against the roof of the mouth on each inhalation. Relax the tongue on the exhalation.

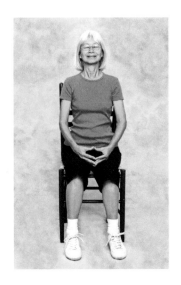

Part Two:

◆ Uncross your feet. Place them flat on the floor.

◆ Touch your fingertips gently together.

◆ With fingertips together, place your hands in your lap.

◆ Focus all your attention on your fingertips. Actually look at your fingertips through closed eyes.

◆ Continue the breathing process described above.

◆ Variation: Do this while standing.

DEEP YAWN (3 MIN)

(from Janet Goodrich)

Why:

More than half of the neurological connections between the brain and the body pass through the jaw joint. The key to whole-body balance and equilibrium can be found in the relationship among proprioceptors in the hips, and feet, and above all the jaw.

Yawning is a natural respiratory reflex that increases circulation to the brain and stimulates the whole body. When you yawn while holding tension points on the jaw, you balance the cranial bones and relax tension in your head and jaw.

Use this activity for increased oxygenation to the brain and eyes, for enhanced verbal and expressive communication, for relaxed vision and thinking during mental work, for reading aloud and public speaking, for deeper vocal resonance and singing, also to improve balance, visual attention, and perception.

How:

◆ Place fingertips on jaw joints.

◆ Pretend to yawn while lightly massaging in front of the joint.

◆ Make a deep, relaxed yawning sound.

◆ Repeat until you begin to make some deep real yawns.

◆ Close your eyes tight when you yawn deeply.

◆ Do until your eyes are watery.

EMOTIONAL STRESS RELEASE (5 MIN)

(from Touch for Health)

Why:

Touching the forehead with the fingers or the flat of the hand allows the brain to experience rational thought. In fact, we do this instinctively whenever we experience major stress. Here's why: in a "fight or flight" response, our brain's activity drops automatically down below, to the limbic system, the brain stem. Directly inside the forehead, though, is the brain center that helps us suppress feelings of anger, frustration, and rage. So when we raise our hands to the forehead, we are inviting the brain to rise to the level of the neocortex—that is, to interpret our experience logically.

Whenever you experience or recall strong mental or emotional stress, lightly hold the ESR (Emotional Stress Release) points, then add a breathing exercise. For example, breathe in, tongue up behind the upper teeth. Then breathe out, tongue down behind the lower teeth. Or just take deep, even breaths. This practice helps to correct a natural but negative response that we all have to stressful experiences, which is to stop breathing.

How:

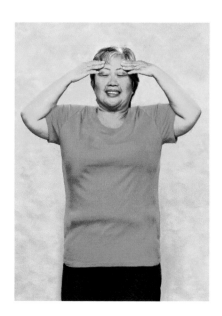

- ◆ Locate the "frontal eminence" on each side of your forehead. This is a protrusion or ridge located directly above the center of the eyebrow and about halfway up to the hairline.

- ◆ Place your fingers gently but firmly on these areas of the forehead.

- ◆ Breathe in, tongue up. Breathe out, tongue down. Or just breathe deeply.

- ◆ Gently but firmly touch the points (do not rub) for about one minute or until you feel relaxed.

- ◆ Variation: A partner can hold these points for you.

Eye Stretches

- Breathe deeply throughout this entire exercise. Do slowly and consciously.
- With head still, look up, deliberately stretching your eye muscles.
- Close your eyes and look up while stretching the eye muscles.
- Look down while stretching your eyes muscles. Do this with your eyes open, then closed.
- Look right, stretching eye muscles with eyes open and then closed.
- Look left, stretching eye muscles with eyes open and then closed.
- Look diagonally up to the right and down to the left. Do with eyes open and closed.
- Look diagonally up to the left, down to the right. Do with eyes open and closed.
- Make clockwise circles with your eyes, then counterclockwise circles. Do with eyes open. Repeat with eyes closed.

Palming

Why:

Soothe and rest your eyes with palming, allowing integration time especially after doing vision movements.

How:

- Rub your hands together to generate heat.
- Close your eyes and cover them with your palms, blocking out the light.
- Breathe deeply.
- Relax.

Eye Acupressure

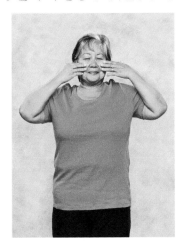

- Gently tap around your eye sockets with your fingertips.
- Push your thumbs into the upper eye sockets on either side of the nose. Press against the inner edges of your eyebrows.
- With thumb and forefinger, squeeze the bridge of your nose.
- With forefingers, push against your cheekbones—the lower eye socket, directly under eyes.

THE GANDHI FAREWELL

(from Carla Hannaford, Ph.D.)

Why:

This easy ritual, the customary way that we end every session, combines sensory integration with spiritual uplift. In a group situation the leader gives each statement and gesture, then the others will echo. Partners can do this together. There's no reason you can't do this solo, too.

How:

♦ "I offer you peace." (hands up, palms facing out)

♦ "I offer you friendship." (hands cupped, in front of you)

♦ "I offer you love." (hands cupped, bring from your heart, moving outward in front of you)

♦ "I hear your needs." (hands cupped around ears)

♦ "I see your beauty." (fingers cover eyes, then uncover eyes)

♦ "I feel your feelings." (arms crisscrossed across chest)

♦ "My power comes from a higher Source." (left hand next to heart, palm facing right; right hand raised above head, palm facing left)

♦ "I honor that Source in you." (bow and namasté, palms together in prayer position)

♦ "Let's work together!" (palms together, fingers interlaced—a fitting symbol of right/left brain integration)

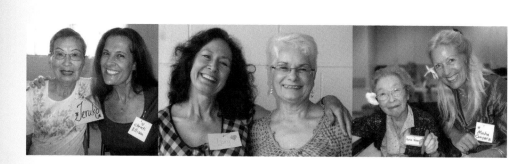

Appendices

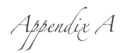

Appendix A

MOVE WITH BALANCE® VIDEO LIST

The book has complete instructions for all the movements: the why and the how. If you are still unsure of a movement or just want to see it in action, please go to www.MoveWithBalance.org. There you will find easy instructions for becoming a member and then viewing the videos. Membership is free to those who bought the book.

The Table of Contents for the videos is arranged similarly to the Table of Contents for the book. Not all the activities have a video, but most of them do. Scroll down to whichever activity you want to view, click, and enjoy.

THE MOVEMENTS

Warm-Ups

Lazy 8s

The Elephant

Arm Activation

The Owl

The Foot Flex

The Gravity Glider

Wake Up

Tune In

Cross-Crawl

Basic Cross Crawl

Cross-Crawl Rap

Infinity Cross-Crawl

You The Dancer

Side Leg-Raise Dancer

Forward Leg-Raise Dancer

Forward Toe-Touch Dancer

Leg-Back Dancer

Side-Lunge Dance

Balls

Solo One-Ball Play

Ball Toss & Bounce

Alternate Ball Toss & Bounce

Ball Toss & Bounce with Clap

Solo Two-Ball Play

Double Ball Toss & Bounce

Alternate Double Ball Toss & Bounce

Partner One-Ball Play

One-Ball Toss & Bounce

Alternate One-Ball Toss & Bounce

Alternate One-Ball Toss & Bounce with Clap

Foot Catch

Partner Two-Ball Play

Double Ball Toss and Catch & Double Ball Bounce and Catch

Alternate Double Ball Toss & Double Ball Bounce and Catch

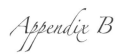

ACTIVITY CARDS

Several of the movements have Activity Cards. You can easily prepare these for your elders or yourself. You can either copy these pages from Appendix B or you can print them off the www.MoveWithBalance.org website. Feel free to use them as is, laminate them, or put them in sheet protectors. You will need Activity Cards for:

SENSORY INTEGRATION:

Clock Face

Slap Tap

Arrows

VISION AND BALANCE:

Vision-Card Balance: Head Moving

Vision-Card Balance: Head Still

SHARPEN YOUR VISION WITH FUSION:

Vision-Card for Pre- and Post-Testing fusion activities

EE Fusion

Inner-Tube Fusion

INSTRUCTIONS:

Clock Face, Slap Tap, and Arrows will be 11 inches high and 8.5 inches wide.

Fold the Vision Card in half so that it is 8.5 inches high and 5.5 inches wide.

Follow directions and cut on the dotted lines for the EE Fusion and Inner-Tube Fusion.

You might want to pick up the cards at the end of each session or give them to the elders.

As our community grows, additional movements that use activity cards will be available in *Move With Balance® II* or on www.MoveWithBalance.org members only section.

Clock Face

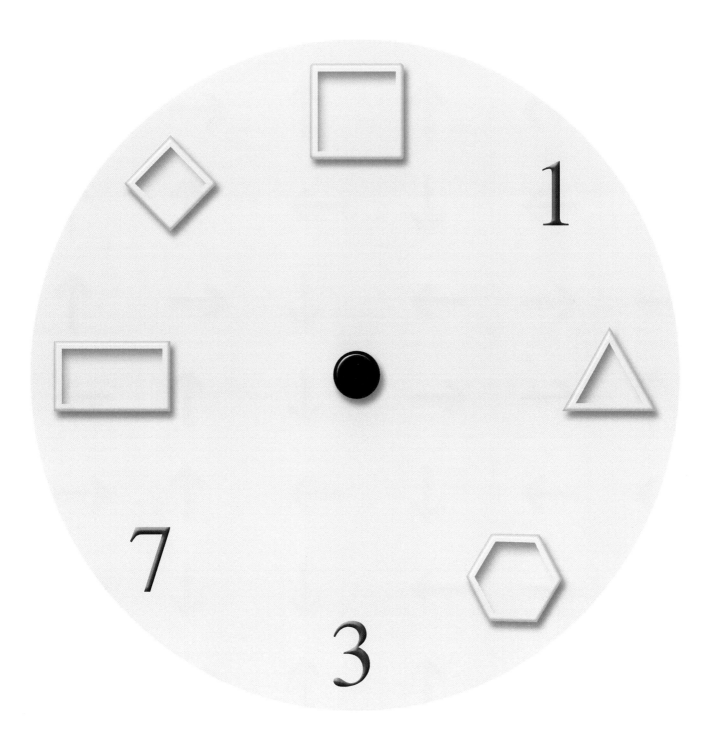

Slap Tap

$L| \quad |R \quad |L \quad R| \qquad |R \quad L| \quad L| \quad R| \quad L|$

$|R \quad L| \quad L| \quad |L \quad R| \quad R| \quad L| \quad |L \quad |R$

$R| \quad |R \quad L| \quad R| \qquad |L \quad L| \quad |L \quad R| \quad R|$

$L| \quad |L \quad R| \quad L| \quad R| \qquad |R \quad |R \quad R| \quad L|$

$|L \quad |R \quad L| \quad R| \qquad |R \quad L| \quad R| \quad L| \quad |L$

$|R \quad L| \quad R| \quad |L \quad |R \quad R| \quad L| \qquad |R \quad R|$

$L| \quad R| \quad R| \quad L| \qquad |L \quad R| \qquad |R \quad L| \qquad |R$

Arrows

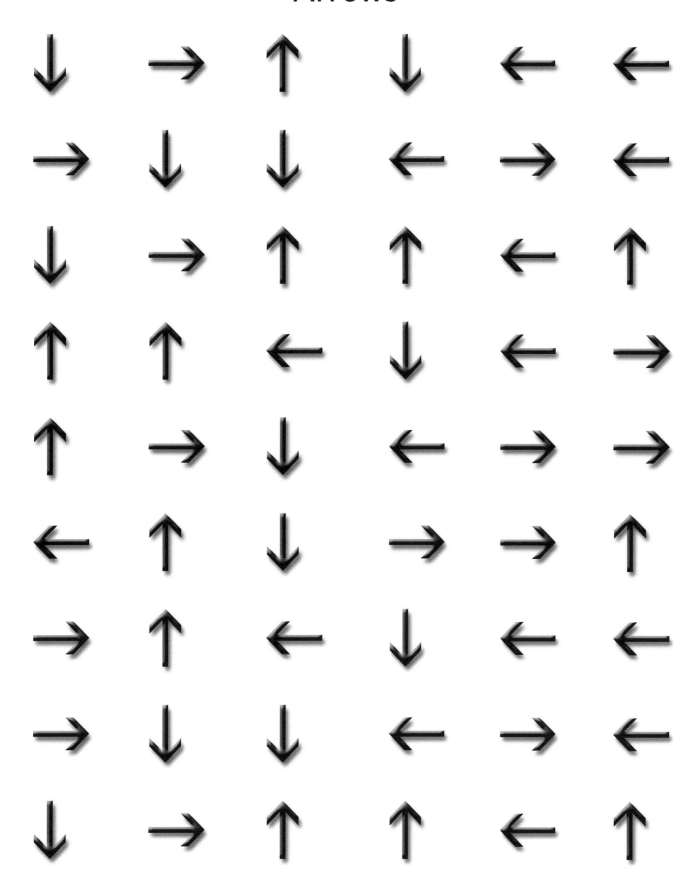

Vision Card

1 I love to see clearly naturally.

2 Natural vision involves every part of me.

3 I breathe and blink easily whenever I use my eyes.

4 Joyful clarity comes when my eyes and mind relax.

5 The feeling of lively and mobile vision is activated when my mental and visual attention stay together.

6 Vivid and colorful visualizations give my wonderful brain the opportunity to practice processing visual input.

7 Delight flows through me when I receive the beautiful colors, textures and contrasts of the natural world through my eyes.

8 When I gaze upon a jewel-toned beetle in my hand, it stimulates my visual system with brilliant shining colors of red, blue, purple and orange.

9 The sunlight shines on the distant hills, the brilliant greens and yellows creating a stunning contrast with the dramatic gray storm clouds.

10 When I allow my attention to stay within this moment, I feel every sense come alive. I love to hear the birds, feel the breeze on my skin and see the movement of trees against the sky.

11 My heart opens as I feel the warmth of the sun at my back, and my eyes receive the joyful colors of a vivid rainbow across the summer sky.

NUCLEAR
CREATE
IMAGE
SEE
OPEN
EYE
COLOR
BEAUTY
FREEDOM

E   E

www.MoveWithBalance.org

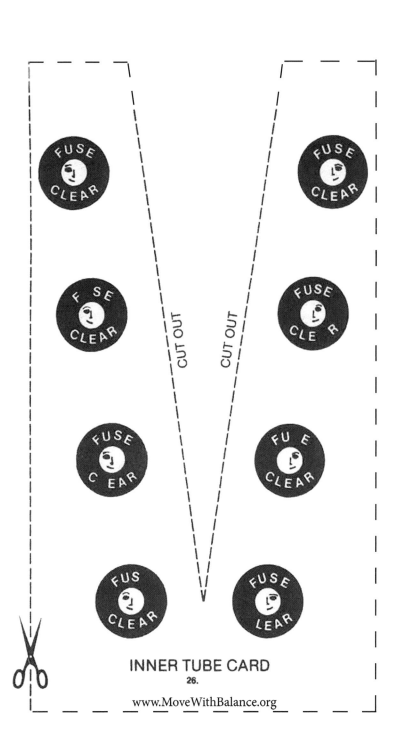

CUT OUT   CUT OUT

INNER TUBE CARD

26.

www.MoveWithBalance.org

Appendix C

SELF-REPORTING TOOLS

Noticing Skills

Whether you are using the program for yourself, working as a caregiver, helping a loved one, or facilitating a group, it is a good idea to sharpen your Noticing Skills. You might want to notice the quality of your balance and your cognitive skills before and after you do the movements. The questions below will guide you so that you become aware of your body and your brain. You do not have to write out answers to all the questions, just explore by sensing and feeling, developing your Noticing Skills, your awareness.

- Balance: Where is your issue? What is your issue? Your weakness, trouble point?

- Sitting: Are you having problems sitting? What are they?

- Standing: Do you have a hard time standing? What happens?

- Walking: Is it hard for you to walk? Describe what happens when you do.

- Sway in each of these dimensions: right/left, up/down, front/back. How do you feel?

- Being present in mind/body: Does your mind wander? How do you feel inside your body?

- Cognitive skills: What is your issue? Your weakness, trouble point?

- Focus/Concentration: Do you have a hard time concentrating or focusing?

- Comprehension—visual, auditory: How is your vision? Your hearing?

- Being present in mind/body: Is it easy for you to think clearly? How is your memory?

- Any other comments: Is there anything else that you notice?

After the movements: Do you notice any changes, improvements?

Move With Balance®   Daily Mental/Physical/Emotional Balance Self-Reporting

Mentee _____ Date _____

This is not a "stop and think" questionnaire. It is to be done quickly, giving the answers that first come into your head. Do at the beginning and end of each session.

1. Before class: circle any words that fit the question. How do you feel before class?

2. After class: block any words that fit the question. How do you feel after class?

tense   calm   quiet   tired   anxious   relaxed   excited   uneasy

worried   peaceful   energized   sleepy   alert   off-balance   sick

troubled   rushed   balanced   clear-headed   lively   scattered

upset   happy   unnerved   up   down   distracted   angry

sad   put-together   grounded in my body   ready to meet my day

Answer the next 2 questions using a scale of 0-5. Zero is feeling your worst & five is best.

1. Before class: Name the number that shows how you are feeling right now. _____

2. After class: Name the number that shows how you are feeling right now. _____

Before class: What movement(s) are you hoping we will do today?

After class: Did the movements meet your expectations? How do you feel?

Any comments?

Move With Balance® Informal Self-Reporting and Evaluation

This form can be filled out by the mentor after observing or discussing the session with the mentee, or by a caregiver, or by an elder doing the program on his/her own. Please adapt this for your needs.

Mentor _____   Week 1   2   3   4   5   6   7   8   9   10 (circle number)

Menteee _____

Informal observations from start to end of session:

1. Emotional state (engagement)

    greatly improved   slightly improved   no improvement

    Comment:

2. Walking — Posture, stance, eyes up, arms, heel-toe, sit-stand, breathing

    greatly improved   slightly improved   no improvement

    Comment:

3. Other comments

Appendix D

THREE INDEPENDENT EVALUATIONS

Evaluation One

Carol S. White, R.N.

May 30, 2008

The Giving Back® Fall Prevention Project [later renamed Move With Balance®], which was recently held at the Kahului Union Church, has demonstrated improvement in the balance activities required for safer sitting, standing, and walking activities of the participant kupuna (elders). Our evaluation of this project utilized evidence-based research methodology. Our findings noted that kupuna reported a reduction in stress and tension and an overall improvement in their mental, physical, and emotional well-being at the conclusion of each session.

Move With Balance® paired senior citizens with mentors previously trained in educational kinesiology and other integrative movements. The pairs in this group worked together on the exercises during weekly sessions over the course of ten weeks.

The most notable findings were:

- Significant increases in the ability of participants to move from sitting to standing without support or with less support than before Move With Balance®.

- Significant increases in the ability of participants to walk using proper posture and needing to look down less than before Move With Balance®.

- Improvements in the attention span/cognition of participants.

- Satisfaction in the mutual engagement and socialization in the Move With Balance® experience expressed by participants and mentors.

Move With Balance® was implemented by Giving Back, a nonprofit organization on Maui whose vision is unite the strengths of senior citizens and trained mentors to improve each other's self-esteem, self-efficacy, and emotional well-being. Move With Balance® was designed specifically to improve physical well-being and cognitive function among our kupuna and to enhance their independence and self-sufficiency in the Maui community.

Carol S. White, R.N.

University of Hawai'i Maui College

Ms. White is an administrative level nurse in community health. She evaluates programs and is responsible for CQI (continuing quality improvement) of the department's patient simulator program.

Evaluation Two
Dr. Lorrin Pang
August 4, 2009

The Giving Back® Fall Prevention Project [later renamed Move With Balance®] was provided to elderly people who attend a senior center on Maui. The Hawai'i Department of Health's Maui office was asked to evaluate the program as close as possible to a cost- benefit format. While there is currently no efficacy data (health cost aversion) for Move With Balance®, another exercise program for elderly Enhanced Fitness shows a twenty percent reduction in medical costs for participants who meet a minimum criteria of attendance. Using standardized fitness tests as a surrogate marker, we showed that Move With Balance® is at a least as efficacious as EF. We assumed that the comparability of fitness markers imply similar averted health costs. Using the observed 76 percent attendance rate and the annual program cost of $28,650 for 38 participants at 5 programs, the annual investment to return ratio was 1:3.4.

The most notable findings were:

- Increases in the ability of participants to move from sitting to standing than before Move With Balance®.

- Increases in the ability of participants to march in place raising the knees to a required height than before Move With Balance®.

- Improvements in the ability to stretch and reach the toes.

- Improvement in ability to reach and touch fingertips behind the back.

- Improvement in the ability to do bicep curls than before Move With Balance®.

- Improvement in the ability to get up from a seated position, walk, turn and return to start.

The Giving Back® Fall Prevention Project was implemented by Giving Back, a nonprofit organization on Maui whose vision is to unite the strengths of trained elder mentors and frail elders to improve each other's strength, flexibility, endurance, balance, coordination, self-esteem, self-efficacy, and emotional well-being. Move With Balance® was designed specifically to improve physical well-being and cognitive functioning among our elders and to enhance their independence and self-sufficiency in the Maui community.

Dr. Lorrin Pang
Director of the Maui District Health Office. The Injury Prevention and Control Program of the Hawai'i State Department of Health requested the evaluation.

Evaluation Three
Dr. Lorrin Pang
Move With Balance® Project
at Roselani Place, Wailuku, Maui
Analysis—June 4, 2012

Summary of Results

Our objective was to compare the number of falls in the group doing the Move With Balance® exercises to the number of falls in those serving as controls (no exercise). We planned for one group to first exercise then become controls and another group to first be controls then exercise.

It became apparent that the first group could not be used subsequently as the control group. There seemed to be a residual effect that continued to reduce falls even after the people in this group stopped the formal exercise program.

Such an outcome is not unusual, as we tend to continue with good habits even after a formal program ends (say, golf lessons or drivers education). We adjusted for this by simply eliminating the first group from ever being used as controls.

Next we noticed that the control and exercise groups may have had very different risks of falling. As a marker for risk of falling we chose the number of falls during the previous year and a half prior to the start of the study. The group exercising had at baseline greater risk of falling. So an adjustment had to be made.

With the two above adjustments there was a statistically significant reduction in falls in the exercise group.

The number of participants is small in this project, but the intriguing findings need to be replicated and expanded for this promising intervention.

The analysis of that project is complete, and has been sent to a publisher for peer review. There was a statistically significant reduction in falls (38% efficacy) in our target group.

Not only are we prepared to rigorously measure outcomes, but our preliminary results look very, very promising. I think Move With Balance® has promise for those with cognitive shortcomings who fall a lot, whether they be in institutions or in homes.

Dr. Lorrin Pang
Director of the Maui District Health Office for the Hawai'i State Department of Health.

Appendix E

MOVEMENT FOR SENIORS: WHY AND HOW MOVE WITH BALANCE® WORKS

by Carla Hannaford, Ph.D.

Biologist and international consultant Dr. Carla Hannaford is the author of *Smart Moves: Why Learning is not All in your Head; The Dominance Factor: How Knowing Your Dominant Eye, Ear, Brain, Hand and Foot Can Improve Your Learning; Awakening the Child Heart: Handbook for Global Parenting;* and *Playing in the Unified Field: Raising and Becoming Conscious, Creative Human Beings.*

Movement is the trademark of all life, and it has finally been recognized as one of the driving forces behind brain growth, learning, and memory throughout our lives.

> *"If we didn't move, we wouldn't need a brain."*
> ~Robert Sylvester

Researchers at the University of California discovered that we can actually grow new nerve cells until the day we die—as many as sixty thousand cells a day in a brain region called the hippocampus, which is our main memory area.[1] Cross-lateral, integrated movements are the key to this cell growth.[2] Recently researchers in Thailand also discovered that new nerve cells were growing in the spinal cord of mice as a result of exercise.[3] Integrated, cross-lateral movements—such as walking, tai chi, yoga, and Brain Gym®— appear to be the key to learning and health for a lifetime.[4]

When we move with balance, we are activating large areas of our brain, including the frontal lobes where our motor cortex resides. These frontal lobes put together the patterns of language, math, complex ideas, and creativity, not to mention the complex emotions of love, altruism, empathy, and compassion. During stress these lobes shut down, as the brain is mostly reacting to save itself. But playful, integrative movements stimulate the motor cortex of the frontal lobes and trigger the production of two important hormones—dopamine and oxytocin. Oxytocin allows us to feel safe and connected. Dopamine sparks our enthusiasm, our motivation to explore and learn, and our ability to move with grace.

The more integrative movements we do, the more whole-brain functions occur, especially in those areas of the frontal lobe which are concerned with memory, emotions, reasoning, will, judgment, personality, and intelligence.

Proof that integrated movement decreases stress—thereby increasing health throughout the body and

---

[1] Kempermann, Gerd & Fred H. Gage. "New Nerve Cells For the Adult Brain," *Scientific American,* May 1999, 48-53.

[2] Van Praag, Henriette, Gerd Kempermann & Fred Gage. "Running Increases Cell Proliferation and Neurogenesis in the Adult Mouse Dentate Gyrus" *Nature Neuroscience,* March 1999 (vol.2:3), 266-270.

[3] Krityakiarana, Win. 2009. "In Brain Research and Instruction," Janet N. Zadina, Ph.D. www.brainresearch.us/sites/default/files/Newsletter%20Spring%202009.pdf(1).

[4] Shaw, Jonathan. "The Deadliest Sin. From survival of the fittest to staying fit just to survive. Scientists probe the benefits of exercise and the dangers of sloth," *Harvard Magazine,* March-April 2004, 36-99.

accommodating optimal learning and memory for a lifetime—was seen in a recent study of a large group of people between age seventy and ninety. Those who danced a couple times a week decreased their chances of Alzheimer's and dementia by 79 percent, and those who played a musical instrument (another integrated cross-lateral movement), decreased their risk by 69 percent.[5]

Those who danced a couple times a week decreased their chances of Alzheimer's and dementia by 79 percent, and those who played a musical instrument (another integrated cross-lateral movement), decreased their risk by 69 percent.

Dancing and playing music require balance, which means activation of the vestibular system, the "entryway to the brain." This area then stimulates the development of the brain stem, especially the cerebellum (which deals with gross motor movement and acts as modulator for almost all functions of the brain), the limbic system (which helps orchestrate our movements in relationship to emotions, sensory input, and memory) and the neo-cortex with its large frontal area or motor cortex. The motor cortex is connected to the proprioceptive area in the sensory cortex, which lets us know what muscles are contracted or relaxed and how to respond in order to move as we want, with flexibility and balance. The vestibular system wakes up the brain so it can easily take in sensory information for optimal learning and memory. Any activity that challenges our sense of balance will help us maintain this important system.

Much of a person's present-day stress comes from immobility. Hours in front of a television or computer screen lead to a loss of balance, a depressed immune system, and an inability to learn and remember. Although stress is a normal part of contemporary living, it is not a normal part of our physiology.

The vestibular system wakes up the brain so it can easily take in sensory information for optimal learning and memory. Any activity that challenges our sense of balance will help us maintain this important system.

The body produces two stress hormones, adrenalin and cortisol, in response to what it perceives as a life-threatening situation. In this "fight-or-flight" state the non-dominant cerebral cortex area will shut down by as much as 85 percent. There is no need for high-level formal reasoning, just reaction. We are unable to think logically or creatively. We can neither learn nor remember easily.[6] However, if we become aware that this has happened and immediately do some simple integrated movement, we can stop the stress reaction in our lives.

Whenever we move in an integrated way (using both sides of the body with balance), we are fully activating whole-brain function. When the whole brain functions in an efficient, integrated way, we can easily see not only the details but also the big picture of a situation. We

[5] Verghese, Joe, et al. "Leisure Activities and the Risk of Dementia in the Elderly," *New England Journal of Medicine*, 2003, vol. 348(25), 2508-2515

[6] Salposky, Robert. *Why Zebras Don't Get Ulcers: An Updated Guide to Stress, Stress-related Diseases, and Coping.* NY: Freeman.1998.

I have found the simple activities of Move With Balance® to have a profound effect on the whole brain/ body system. Plus, the fun of doing them raises the levels of neuro-chemicals that optimize all learning and increase our quality of life.

take on have a balanced physical structure that can accommodate the movements we need at the moment. Best of all, we connect with other people in empathetic, altruistic ways.

I have found the simple activities of Move With Balance® to have a profound effect on the whole brain/body system. Plus, the fun of doing them raises the levels of neuro-chemicals that optimize all learning and increase our quality of life.

These integrated movements require balance, and so they activate the vestibular system—especially if they are done slowly while standing up. Also, most of the movements are cross-lateral, which means that they activate both the motor cortex (in the frontal lobes) and the sensory cortex (in the parietal lobes) of both hemispheres. They give us access to the big picture and the details of our life.

Specific Activities and How They Work

Connecting the Circuits

Dr. Wayne Cook created what Move With Balance® calls "Connecting the Circuits." This activates huge areas of the neocortex having to do with every part of our body. Since this activity requires the complex movement of both hands, just as with knitting, crocheting, typing, or playing a musical instrument, we are activating large areas of the sensory/motor cortexes of both hemispheres. Since the exercise makes us stand and cross one leg over the other, it is one of our most cross-lateral movements. Because it requires balance, it activates the vestibular system.

Tune In

Tune In, a simple Touch for Health exercise, activates 140 points in the ear. These points connect directly to other points throughout the body via the meridian system. (Anyone skeptical of acupuncture should know that the National Medical Library in Washington DC accepts over sixty journals each month on the subject of traditional Chinese medicine. Every such publication validates the existence of a complex meridian system throughout the body.) Because it activates the ears to become alert, Tune In assists memory. Hearing and smelling are our first channels into memory.

Deep Yawn

Deep Yawn from the Janet Goodrich Method has been found to relax all the areas of the face and hands. Moreover, it stimulates all the nerves that cross the temporal-mandibular joint, thus increasing our ability to see, hear, and communicate. Yawning has been found to increase alertness and concentration. It optimizes brain activity and metabolism, improves cognitive function, increases memory recall, lowers stress, relaxes every part of the body, and improves voluntary muscle control.[7]

THE LAZY 8S

The Lazy 8s, otherwise known as Infinity Signs, assist both near and far focus. They ease writing and communication. Since both hands are being used to direct the eyes, large areas of the motor and sensory cortexes of both hemispheres are being used. So are the visual cortexes in the occipital lobes. As the eyes move in this infinity pattern, the six big external eye muscles get used equally. Thus those muscles are strengthened and the eyes are trained to team together for better vision. Focusing on different distances strengthens the inner eye muscles, which work the lens of the eye to accommodate for near and far vision.

When Lazy 8s are used for writing, they allow the muscles of the hand to relax in an even flow. They increase hand-eye coordination and our ability to communicate ideas coherently. Whenever I have "writer's block," I do Lazy 8s and the ideas again begin to flow.

WAKE UP

The Wake Up exercise has us holding the navel, thus bringing attention to our center of gravity. This simple posture activates the vestibular system and wakes the brain to incoming information. We also hold the 27th points on the kidney meridian, which has been recognized for centuries as being connected with heart and lung function. Touching these points brings more oxygen to the brain for clearer thought.

YOU THE DANCER

Athletes use the Leg-Back Dancer exercise to release tension in the back of the legs, sacrum, and neck so that they can move with more flow and balance. Here's why: stress triggers the tendon guard reflex, which causes the back of the knees to lock. That's good in a fight-or-flight situation because no matter which option we choose, we won't tear the Achilles tendon. But now, because the knees are locked, the balance is thrown forward on the balls of the feet, or else back on the heels. This teetering in the body causes the back and neck muscles to tighten so that we don't fall over. If stress is chronic, this tightening of the back and neck muscles can cause slipped discs and major back and neck problems. By doing the Leg-Back Dancer, we are giving the message to the muscles to relax, not just behind the knees but all through the back and neck.

The Footflex does the same thing as the Leg-Back Dancer. When we hold the Achilles tendon and tendons behind the knee, we give a message to calf muscles—relax, release the tendon guard reflex.

The Side-Lunge Dancer works with the iliopsis or psoas muscles that enable us to bend over or to raise

---

[7] Newberg, Andrew & Mark Robert Waldman. *Breakthrough Finds from a Leading Neuroscientist, How God Changes Your Brain.* 155-159

our legs. When we are stressed, the psoas muscle tends to tighten, causing us to be stiff and inflexible in our movements. The Side-Lunge Dancer activity tells the psoas muscle to relax. We become flexible and better at regaining our balance.

ARM ACTIVATION

The Arm Activation works with the muscles of the upper back (trapezius, latissimus dorsi, rhomboid, scalene) that connect into the armpit area. These muscles tighten when we are under stress. That tightening causes frozen shoulders and the inability to move the arms in a large circle around the side of the body. This movement helps release the tension in the muscles so that the shoulder can relax and move freely.

THE OWL

This activity also works to release the tendon guard reflex. By strongly holding the trapezius and allowing the head to fall forward, we can feel the muscles of the neck release and relax as the head moves from side to side.

THE GRAVITY GLIDER

The Gravity Glider also assists in releasing the tendon guard reflex in the back of the legs, also tension in the back and neck. It tells the muscles and ligaments to relax. As we relax into this movement, all the muscle release their tension. The body lengthens in response.

THE ELEPHANT

The Elephant is one of the most integrative of the Move With Balance® activities. First, by flexing the knees we relax the tendon guard reflex. Then by laying the ear on the shoulder, we release the trapezius muscle on the opposite side and stimulate the semicircular canals of the inner ear, thus activating the vestibular system. Then with the arm extended and the eyes following the Lazy 8 movement of the arm, using a fluid up-and-down movement of the body that releases the psoas muscle, the whole body becomes involved in integration. This movement comes from the core of the body (around the navel). Thus it integrates early reflexes and encourages the body to be very balanced and alert.

CROSS-CRAWL

The Cross-Crawl is simply a conscious walking action. Health professionals constantly affirm that walking is important for the whole body. Walking is considered the number-one exercise for everyone—it does not stress the system, it integrates both the right and left sides of the body, and it assists with balance and strengthens our muscles and ligaments.

All these Move With Balance® activities help you grow new nerve cells and stay flexible, alert, and balanced. These are passionate, playful movements and rich sensory experiences that anchor thought, build mental agility, and encourage life-long learning. After all, our brain cells communicate in response to movement, sensory input, and a sense of safety.

Carla Hannaford, Ph.D.
www.GreatRiverBooks.com

Appendix F

BRAIN PROCESSES AFFECTED BY MOVE WITH BALANCE®

Commentary by

Louis Weissman

President, Human Performance Group, LLC

global providers of the Learning Breakthrough Program™

Website: www.Learningbreakthrough.com

Note: We have adapted the following explanations from a longer essay by Louis Weissman. With his permission we have added some statements that make the connection between general science and the movements described in this manual. We are sincerely grateful to Mr. Weissman. –MWB

BALANCE

The vestibular system—in other words, our sense of balance—plays a central role in the biological functioning of all of the brain's activity. As a child grows in the womb, the vestibular system becomes the first set of structures and "sense" to develop. It serves as the fundamental organizational tool for the development of all the other brain processes.

Our model of the world is in three-dimensional space with a clear sense of up and down. Other major brain systems—motor, tactile, auditory, and visual—develop in relation to the vestibular system, or sense of balance.

Because the vestibular system plays such a key role in the foundations of perception, balance problems can cause many seemingly unrelated problems in brain function.

SENSORY/MOTOR INTEGRATION

Mobility and balance depend upon three types of sensory information to the brain: visual input; head positioning information from the inner ear; and a sense of spatial orientation from specialized receptor cells found in the skin, muscles, joints, and tendons.

Our three-dimensional model of the world provides the framework into which all other sensory data must be integrated. Because the vestibular system is the basis of this three-dimensional model, it governs the effectiveness of communication between the senses and the brain. Otherwise, each sensory input is independent of the other. For instance, your sense of spatial orientation (proprioception) is independent of vision.

Move With Balance® helps people improve cognitive functions and balance by improving the way information is transmitted between different sensory centers in the brain, all of which rely fundamentally on the sense of balance.

Spatial Awareness

Spatial awareness is the organized perception, tracking, and monitoring of the objects in the space around us as well as our body's position in space. It is another fundamental brain function that informs all higher-level cognitive activities.

Spatial awareness requires that we have a model of the three-dimensional space around us, and it requires us to integrate information from all of our senses. Because spatial awareness is so important in all activities of human life, deficiencies in spatial awareness can hold people back from achieving their true potential. However, activities that refine the vestibular system and develop sensory integration help refine spatial awareness and all aspects of brain processing.

Integration of the Left and Right Hemispheres of the Brain

The human brain is composed of two hemispheres that function like two networked computers. The left hemisphere receives motor and sensory input from the right side of the body and the right hemisphere receives input from the left side. When we bring the two systems together and begin the task of developing harmony and synchrony, the first step is to achieve an efficient balance between the operations taking place in the two sides of the brain.

Most mental processes involve both sides of the brain. Therefore, integration problems between the two hemispheres can result in inefficiencies in brain processes. Weak integration between the two sides of the brain can lead to a vicious cycle. For example, a person may suppress one eye (corresponding to one side of the brain). This means that the person reads with one eye only, the "strong eye." As a result, the brain networks used to support the "weak" eye will become further disorganized through lack of use, exacerbating the initial lack of integration.

Since the left controls right and vice-versa, a person can refine the integration between the two sides of the brain through activities involving both sides of the body.

When we learn to crawl, we establish a synchronized cross patterning. Both sides of the body and both hemispheres of the brain start operating under the control of a consistent timing system. Both sides of the body are matched perfectly. Both sides of the brain are in phase.

As the child learn to walk, the sensory integration and balance requirements increase. In order to achieve synchrony the child must achieve a higher level of integration between the two hemispheres of the brain. The most efficient possible walking pattern for a human being is the one in which the two arms are swinging as pendulums counterbalancing the movement of the legs and setting the rhythmic pace for the total movement pattern.

Successful integration between the two sides of the brain is necessary for improving all brain processes including those for motor skills, physical coordination, and all other higher-order cognitive processes. The Move With Balance® activities improve this hemispheric integration.

BRAIN TIMING AND REACTION TIMES

Successful integration of the two hemispheres of the brain cannot be accomplished without efficient brain timing. The greater the balance requirements, the faster the brain must process information provided by the senses and the two hemispheres of the brain.

When we watch people move, we are indirectly observing the efficiency of brain processing. Suppressions, rigidity, and uncoordinated movements are the result of bad timing and faulty integration. They indicate poor brain processing ability that can manifest itself as learning problems. However, poor brain timing is improved by activities that require the individual to move both sides of the body. Such activities run throughout the Move With Balance® program.

SEQUENCING

Individuals must be able to construct complex patterns in order to carry out multi-step activities. Those with motor-skill deficiencies and poor coordination suffer from a limited ability to sequence. Conversely, improvements in motor-skill efficiency and brain timing have positive effects on basic sequencing. Activities that address the inefficiencies in the neural networks can be very helpful in changing the physiological conditions in the brain that contribute to this problem.

BINOCULAR EYE TEAMING

Binocular teaming is the ability of both eyes to work together. Binocularity—the working together of the two eyes to provide different views that the brain then integrates into one image—is an important visual processing skill. It is responsible for providing depth perception. We need it in order to perform a variety of visual tasks such as tracking, fixating, converging, and visual motor integration.

The eyes are only part of the brain process we call "vision." The vestibular system is just as critical and is tightly integrated with the eyes. If the eyes don't team well, problems arise that adversely affect the sense of balance. This is why Move With Balance® is designed with products and activities that make demands on the brain in terms of balance while simultaneously stimulating the visual system to improve binocular teaming and visual processing.

PROPRIOCEPTION

The brain constantly engages in a process designed to position the body based on the information it receives from our senses. This process is called proprioception—the awareness of movement and body position. Think of it as the body's joint and muscle positioning system. Proprioception depends on the brain's ability to integrate information from all the senses, the muscles and joints, and the vestibular system.

Proprioception allows you to close your eyes and lift your arm and still know which way your palm is turned. It informs you of where you are and where you belong in space.

Many experts assert that a reduced sense of proprioception is the primary cause of age-related falls. Sensitivity to the receptor cells that tell the brain where you are in space tends to decrease as you age. The brain misses these messages about our posture and positioning, causing loss of balance.

Balance activities that integrate the visual, auditory, kinesthetic, tactile and vestibular senses have the effect of improving the proprioceptive processes that help to reduce injuries and improve performance. As neural capability and efficiency increases, a variety of other benefits are realized. Timing improves, vision improves, sense of balance improves, mental processing improves, reaction time improves, proprioception improves. This is obviously of great importance for seniors. Move With Balance® provides a system that improves cognitive functions and physical performance at the same time.

THE PROGRESSIVE CHALLENGE

As the difficulty of an activity increases, the brain must grow new neurons and dendrites in order to rise to the challenge. This is why the difficulty level of these Move With Balance® activities should keep increasing over time.

If a person has difficulty executing a particular activity, this may be because the activity's challenge exceeds his or her brain's current capabilities. To avoid a sense of failure, everyone should start out with activities that are simple enough to perform and gradually increase the difficulty level. As the difficulty level increases, the required spatial awareness, brain hemisphere integration, and brain-timing precision will increase along with it.

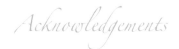
Acknowledgements

There are so many people I want to acknowledge—people I have studied with, people I have worked with, people who have been part of this replication project, people for whom I have taught, board members, mentors, and grantors. I thank those and many more for being part of my life as this project has unfolded and continues to unfold.

In particular I want to acknowledge those people who contributed in large and small ways to the thinking and activities set forth in this manual.

I have been a Licensed Brain Gym® Instructor since 1986. The Brain Gym® movements and exercises used in this book or product are used with the permission of Brain Gym® International but do not particularly reflect the educational philosophy of Brain Gym® International nor the Brain Gym® founders, Paul and Gail Dennison, California, USA. Educational Kinesiology Foundation www.braingym.org

In 1989 I became a certified Touch for Health instructor. This is some of the simplest and most profound work I have ever experienced. Matthew Thie, M. Ed., was so happy that I was going to use some Touch for Health exercises in this book. He told me it was just what his father John, the founder of Touch for Health, wanted—to make the exercises widely available to many people. www.touch4health.com.

Dr. Wayne Cook, a pioneer in energy medicine and bioenergetics, created the "Connect the Circuits" exercise. Also known as the Wayne Cook Posture, it restores balance whether we are over-energized or under-energized. Brain Gym® and Touch for Health both use it. They call it "Cook's Hookups." Leonardo da Vinci said, "Movement is the source and cause of all life." We are moving and balancing energy with the Wayne Cook Posture.

Victoria Tennant created the "rap" poem to go along with the cross-crawl. Her clever rhymes are perfect for increasing the challenge of the cross-crawl. Victoria Tennant Consulting. www.victoriatennantconsulting.com

Edvin Manniko O.D. is a vision-training/behavioral optometrist. I was lucky enough to do vision training with Dr. Ed Manniko's clients in Denver, Colorado. We used balls, beanbags, balance boards, rebounders, and much more in our exercises. Many of the ball and beanbag exercises are based on what I learned from him. Dr. Manniko has conducted extensive research in the area of visual enhancement, and he has established a diverse clientele consisting of world-class athletes, students, learning-disabled individuals, and injury victims. For the past twenty years every time I have returned to Denver, I have visited him and learned something new. To learn more about his excellent work, seek out Accelerated Visual Performance, LLC info@opticdynamics.com

Jon Bredal taught me "Row Your Boat" in his Balancing the Child class. Currently he has a Heal the Child Program, which includes working with children and their families using lots integrative games. www.JonBredal.org.

I learned the "Rock Paper Scissors, Cock Hen Chick" game in a Five Animal Play class from Amy Choi and Conrad Ho. It is based on the Rock Paper Scissors game that we all played as children. Amy and Conrad use many traditional Chinese games and animal movements in their practice. I modified their game somewhat for the elders. Brain Body Centre, Ltd, http://www.brainbodycentre.com

Vision training/behavioral optometrist Bobbie Dirks, Lyn Wilson, and I founded the Learning Hui, Makawao, Maui, Hawai'i in 2000. We have worked with children of all ages (K-12) and abilities to enhance their learning, perception, and sensory integration. It was Bobbie who introduced me to Clock Face and Slap Tap.

I became a Certified Natural Vision Improvement Instructor with Janet Goodrich in 1987 in Australia, and I have used her methods ever since. Janet inspired the activity that I call the "Deep Yawn." She would have us yawn for twenty minutes straight in her certification classes. Also, the Vision Card comes from my training with Janet. Her daughter Carina has carried on Janet's work, The Janet Goodrich Method, www.JanetGoodrichMethod.com

Dr. Edward Friedman wrote a wonderful book called *Dr. Friedman's Vision Training Program*. I have been using this book since 1987, and it seems it's time for a new copy as this one is really ragged. I use "Inner Tubes" from his book to practice fusion.

There are so many others I want to acknowledge and thank. For example, Carla Hannaford, Ph.D., for her inspiring classes, books, love, and support. Also, Peggy Sanches for being with me throughout this adventure as a mentor, as a board member, and as my sounding-board/brainstorming friend. Peggy has won the Senior Citizen Volunteer Award from the State of Hawai'i twice now (2008 and 2012) for her work as a Giving Back volunteer. She won the AARP Volunteer from Hawai'i in December 2012.

I must acknowledge the mentors Eloise "Elo" Shak, Theodore "Theo" Trouerbach, and Yvonne "Bonnie" Gaspar, who acted as the models for this book. And I'm thinking of all the volunteers who worked over the years in Move With Balance®, giving their love and dedication to the frail elders and children they mentored. I thank everyone who has been a board member for Giving Back throughout the years. I appreciate all you have done to make this project a reality.

James Mylenek tirelessly assisted me in this project. Lorrin Pang M.D. and Carol White R.N. provided their expertise in researching the program with their independent evaluations. I acknowledge my editor Paul Wood, who helps me write "so that the man or woman on the street will understand what you are trying to say."

Leola Muromoto and Dana Acosta of Kaunoa Senior Services, a wonderful program and facility maintained by the County of Maui, took a chance on me and allowed me to work with their seniors and develop Move With Balance® during the past eighteen years. I thank all the grantors who contributed to Giving Back, especially the Island Innovation Fund.

Each and every one of you matters and is significant in the forward movement of Move With Balance®. You helped this program to be where it is today.

The inspiration for Giving Back was my grandmother Gammy, who loved and accepted me for who I am. Our intergenerational bond grew as she mentored me, with the end result being Giving Back® and its community-building intergenerational programs.

Mahalo (thank you) to all of these and many more.

Karen Peterson